OUTCOME MEASURES
for HEALTH EDUCATION
and other
HEALTH CARE INTERVENTIONS

OUTCOME MEASURES
for HEALTH EDUCATION
and other
HEALTH CARE INTERVENTIONS

Kate Lorig

Anita Stewart

Philip Ritter

Virginia González

Diana Laurent

John Lynch

SAGE Publications
International Educational and Professional Publisher
Thousand Oaks London New Delhi

For information address:

 SAGE Publications, Inc.
2455 Teller Road
Thousand Oaks, California 91320
E-mail: order@sagepub.com

SAGE Publications Ltd.
6 Bonhill Street
London EC2A 4PU
United Kingdom

SAGE Publications India Pvt. Ltd.
M-32 Market
Greater Kailash I
New Delhi 110 048 India

Printed in the United States of America

Library of Congress Cataloging-in-Publication Data

Main entry under title:

Outcome measures for health education and other health care
  interventions / Kate Lorig ... [et al.].
     p. cm.
  Includes bibliographical references and index.
  ISBN 0-7619-0066-7 (acid-free paper). — ISBN 0-7619-0067-5 (pbk.:
  acid-free paper)
  1. Health education—Evaluation. 2. Medical care—Evaluation.
  I. Lorig, Kate.
  RA440.5.O94 1996
  613—dc20   95-50181

This book is printed on acid-free paper.

     97 98 99   10 9 8 7 6 5 4 3

Sage Production Editor: Vicki Baker
Sage Cover Designer: Candice Harman
Sage Typesetter: Danielle Dillahunt

Contents

Acknowledgments

Many people and organizations were instrumental in the completion of this book. The Chronic Disease Self-Management Program is a collaborative research study conducted by the Stanford University School of Medicine and the Kaiser Permanente Medical Care Program, Northern California. The study was funded by California Tobacco-Related Disease Research Program Award No. RT156 and the Agency for Health Services Policy and Research Grant No. 5RO1HS06680. The validation of the Spanish scales was funded by the National Institute for Nursing Research Grant No. R01 NRO3146-01. We owe many thanks to these agencies and particularly our program officers. Without these awards, this work would not have been possible.

Others to whom we owe a debt of gratitude are David Sobel, Halsted Holman, Albert Bandura, Dan Bloch, and William Byron Brown, Jr. All have collaborated and added their wisdom to this work. Roslyn Bienenstock spent many hours securing all the necessary permissions to reprint instruments. Christine Smedley and Vicki Baker from Sage Publications have been ever helpful with their suggestions. Cielo Santos and Larissa Ortiz spent many hours in data coding and entry and typing manuscripts.

Finally, we would like to thank the more than 1,500 people who have completed our questionnaires.

Introduction

Before the mid-1970s, most health care interventions were evaluated on the basis of their effects on physiologic outcomes, such as blood pressure and blood glucose; clinical outcomes, such as prognosis; or mortality. At the same time, health education interventions were evaluated primarily on the basis of changes in knowledge or behaviors. Since that time, health services, behavioral medicine, and health education interventions have added outcomes based on patients' perspective of their day-to-day functioning and well-being. These more recent outcomes fall into several categories: physical disability (such as limitations in activities of daily living and role limitations), mental distress (such as depression and anxiety), distressful symptoms (such as pain and shortness of breath), and cost, which is often measured by surrogates such as utilization of health care resources.

As assessment of health outcomes from the patient's perspective has become the new standard, many instruments (scales) have been developed. For the most part these are self-administered, which has allowed for more practical and relatively low-cost evaluations.

Based on the above trends in outcomes measurement, this book presents a collection of outcome measures with strong psychometric properties that can be used by practitioners and researchers to evaluate a variety of intervention studies, with a special emphasis on health education interventions.

The emphasis of the book is on a set of outcome measures that were developed at the Stanford Patient Education Research Center for use in its studies of chronic disease self-management programs. Because most of these scales have not been previously published, we also present how the scales were formulated and the psychometric properties of each scale. In addition, we present in the appendices several scales formulated by other researchers that we and our colleagues have found useful.

Chapter 1 contains information on the rationale for the Chronic Disease Self-Management (CDSM) study instruments and how we determined which outcomes to measure. Chapter 2 contains psychometric information on each of the scales used in the study. Appendix A contains the actual items in each of the study scales, along with information about coding. Please note that our scales in Appendix A can be used without further copyright permission. But if they are used, we would like to be informed of study results and any problems that may arise in the use of these instruments. Please send your results or queries to the Stanford Patient Education Research Center, 1000 Welch Road, Suite 204, Palo Alto, CA 94304, or contact us by e-mail at KRL@DBN.Stanford.edu.

Appendixes B through E are compendiums of outcome instruments that we have collected from other sources. For each instrument, we give references and coding information. In Appendix F, we present Spanish translations for some of the instruments. These translations were part of a study evaluating a Spanish Arthritis Self-Management Program. The information on the development and psychometric properties of these instruments is referenced. It should be noted that the development process included Spanish-speaking people from different countries of origin. These translations use "standard" Spanish, which should be understood by most Spanish-speaking people in the United States, Mexico, and Central and South America. Finally, we provide a list of additional sources for more measures in Appendix G.

The scales in this book do not represent a comprehensive collection of all appropriate outcome measures. Nor are they meant to represent the "best" measures. Rather, they were chosen because they have all been used by or are well known to the authors. They have proven themselves to be understood by, and acceptable to, patients and other research subjects. Nearly all of them have proven useful in measuring change in intervention studies.

Conceptual Basis for the Chronic Disease Self-Management Study

In the past century, the human life span has increased by almost 30 years. A child born in 1991 can expect to live approximately 76 years, whereas a child born in 1900 was expected to live to only 47 (U.S. Dept. of Health and Human Services, 1994). The aging of the population is perhaps the most dominant demographic feature of the late 20th century. The number of persons aged 65 and over in the United States has grown from 3.1 million in 1900 (4% of the population) to more than 30 million today (12% of the population) (U.S. Senate Special Committee on Aging, 1988). Projections for the future suggest that by the year 2000 there will be 39 million elderly (age 65 and over) and that by the year 2020 there will be 52 million elderly. By the year 2030, 22% of the U.S. population will be elderly.

Chronic disease is often a characteristic of aging. People 60 years of age and above have on average slightly more than two chronic conditions, the most common being hypertension, arthritis, cardiovascular disease, and lung disease (Clark et al., 1991). Rothenberg and Koplan (1990) have shown that the prevalence of 15 out of 16 chronic conditions increased in the period from 1960 to 1980. Some diseases, such as diabetes, chronic obstructive pulmonary disease, and arthritis, have increased by as much as 100%. Thus, overall, the morbidity and disability associated with these conditions have increased.

The last 15 years have witnessed a change in the way our society views aging. Growing old is no longer thought of as the end of the productive period of life and as a time of inevitable decline in physical and mental health. Rather, terms such as *successful aging, productive aging, robust aging,* and the *compression of morbidity* (Butler & Gleason, 1985; Fries, 1980; Katz, 1983; Rowe & Kahn, 1987) are being used in literature. We have mounting evidence that lifestyle in terms of nutrition, exercise, and smoking, among other behaviors, can prevent or delay chronic conditions and can also improve these conditions or slow deterioration once they occur. Thus, naturally occurring behaviors and health practices as well as interventions to improve lifestyle behaviors can potentially enhance social functioning, improve physical and mental health, prolong independent living, and promote greater autonomy.

Despite the recognition that learning to live with chronic diseases may well be one of the most important developmental tasks of aging, neither medical care nor health education has had much to offer people with chronic diseases. For example, medical care is limited in its ability to relieve symptoms or reverse disease processes of chronic disease. The educational programs that do exist fall roughly into three categories: (a) prevention, (b) wellness, and (c) disease-specific programs. Prevention programs are aimed at removing the root causes of disease through broad based interventions that offer immunizations, modification of personal behavior or reduction of the environmental causes of disease. Wellness programs attempt to maintain or improve levels of physical and psychological functioning in healthy populations. They generally assume the absence of chronic conditions. Disease-specific programs focus on only one particular disease, with little or no consideration of how chronic conditions interact or how program recommendations may be impossible to follow because of existing comorbidities. For example, someone in cardiac rehabilitation may have a difficult time exercising because of osteoarthritis of the knees or hips.

These four factors: an aging population, an increase in both chronic disease and comorbidity, new concepts about aging, and the lack of health education programs appropriate for persons with multiple chronic conditions, served as the impetus for the Chronic Disease Self-Management Study.

The aims of the Chronic Disease Self-Management Program were

1. To create a program that could address concerns of persons with a variety of chronic conditions
2. To evaluate this program in terms of changes in behavior, health status, and health care utilization
3. To explore the role of self-efficacy, or one's confidence, in facilitating improvements in health status and reductions in health care utilization

The philosophy behind the program is that tertiary prevention efforts should be guided by the concept of living with and dying with (rather than dying from) chronic diseases. By delaying disability and reducing the toll of suffering and limitations, self-management programs have the potential for improving quality of life and reducing health care costs. Several researchers have shown that prevention programs for older adults can indeed be successful in prolonging the period of optimal physical functioning, maintaining mental functioning and social activity, minimizing disability and discomfort, preparing for retirement, and supporting people faced with terminal illness (Breslow & Somers, 1988; Omenn, 1990).

To create such a program, and the appropriate evaluation instruments, it is first necessary to identify common problems faced by patients with various chronic diseases, common health behaviors that can ameliorate the adverse impact of those diseases, and appropriate health status outcomes that can be affected by the intervention. This was accomplished by four types of investigation: (a) impressions gathered from prior experience with studies of this type, (b) a literature review, (c) a series of focus groups with older people with different chronic conditions, and (d) a review of social psychological theory. Below we examine each of these areas more closely.

Prior Experience ■

The idea of a self-management intervention to address issues of chronic disease evolved from the knowledge and experiences gained over 12 years in conducting a community-based education program for people with arthritis (Lorig & González, 1992; Lorig & Holman, 1993). These earlier arthritis programs were evaluated in terms of health behaviors, patient-reported health status, and health care utilization.

The arthritis self-management studies found that participants on average reduced their pain and utilization of health care providers, although no changes in disability were observed. These changes persisted for up to 4 years (Lorig, Seleznick, et al., 1989). In work conducted by Lenker and colleagues, it was found that improvements in health status were associated more with increased self-efficacy than with adoption of new health behaviors (Lenker, Lorig, & Gallagher, 1984). This finding led to further exploration of the role of self-efficacy in reducing pain. This is discussed further in the following section on theory.

Health education researchers at the Stanford Arthritis Center also observed that many of the patients enrolled in their programs were dealing with a variety of other chronic diseases. Patients often reported improvement in these other conditions, although they were not specifically addressed by the arthritis intervention. These experiences led to two general impressions about chronic diseases and older persons:

1. Different chronic diseases often cause similar problems related to activities of daily living, interactions with the health care system, communication with family and friends, and dealing with negative emotions such as fear, anxiety and depression.
2. Many older people are willing and able to better self-manage their chronic disease(s) when they are given appropriate instruction.

Literature Review ■

A review of patient education and self-care literature identified 12 self-management tasks which were common across chronic conditions (Clark et al., 1991). These tasks included (a) recognizing and responding to symptoms, including monitoring symptoms and controlling triggers to symptoms; (b) using medications; (c) managing acute episodes and emergencies; (d) maintaining good nutrition and an appropriate diet; (e) maintaining adequate exercise and physical activity; (f) not smoking; (g) using relaxation and stress-reducing techniques; (h) interacting appropriately with health care providers; (i) seeking information and using community resources; (j) adapting work and other role functions; (k) communicating with significant others; and (l) managing the negative emotions and psychological responses to illness. The reviewers suggested that it may be "possible to identify and elaborate a common set of tasks that patients, regardless of disease and comorbidities, need to undertake to successfully self-manage" (p. 23). They also suggested further study of this possibility.

■ Focus Groups

A qualitative needs assessment using focus groups was conducted to ensure that the program was sensitive to the issues faced by those with multiple chronic conditions. Focus groups are semistructured interviews in which groups of 8 to 12 people openly discuss ideas introduced by a moderator (Basch, 1987; Morgan, 1988).

Eleven focus groups were held in various community settings, including senior centers, community centers, health maintenance organizations, and voluntary health agencies. Participants included both "well elders" and people with heart disease, lung disease, stroke, or arthritis. Participants were invited to (a) describe their diseases and what they thought caused them; (b) explain their feelings and beliefs about getting older; (c) describe the physical, social, and emotional impacts of chronic disease on their lives and the lives of their families; (d) tell how they coped with the problems caused by their disease; and (e) elaborate on their fears, hopes, and wishes for the future. Each group's discussion was tape recorded and later transcribed to provide verbatim accounts of the session.

During the second stage of the needs assessment, the transcripts were coded and categorized. On the basis of the actual discussions, the categories did not exactly match the questions. The investigator who conducted the groups began by reading the transcripts and arriving at a preliminary list of themes for each topic. In addition, one randomly selected transcript was read by four other reviewers, who also selected themes. Then all five reviewers met to compare and justify their list of themes and decide on a final list of themes.

The third stage involved coding the transcripts according to the final list of themes. If a focus group statement contained more than one idea or was not clear, multiple codes could be used. The themes were examined with the aid of Ethnograph software (Seidel, Friese, & Leonard, 1995). This program enabled all the statements made by focus group members that related to a specific theme to be grouped and recalled together. For example, all the statements that individuals had made concerning the physical impacts of disease could be retrieved as one group. Once the statements had been grouped according to themes, they were again examined by the review panel to ensure the consistency of the statements relating to each theme. If statements were not consistent, they were recoded. (Table 1.1 gives a summary of the final list of themes.)

The statements from the focus groups were very useful in clarifying issues and problems that are not usually considered in designing patient education interventions. These included such topics as coping with anger and maintaining role functions in the face of progressive chronic illness. The transcripts also provided the actual terminology and phrasing that people used when talking about dealing

TABLE 1.1 Theme Categories Derived From the Focus Groups

Disease Causation	**Disease Impacts**
Stress	Determination to overcome the problems
Lifestyle	Physical limitation
Fate/luck	Depression
Heredity	Lack of control of symptoms and of one's
Exercise	life
Smoking	Sleep
Other psychological constructs	Fatalism about the future
Aging	Anxiety
Loss of:	Body awareness
Family/social contact	Acceptance of limitations
Self-esteem	Family/friends relationships
Independence	**Future Concerns**
Physical ability	Family/friends relationships
Mental ability	Death
Role competence	Disability/loss of independence
Confidence	Accommodations/housing
Feelings of:	Communication with family
Acceptance	Future planning
Anger	Finance
Helplessness	Emotional support
Frustration	Uncertainty
Opportunity/enjoyment	Memory loss
Denial	**Health Service Utilization**
	Satisfaction
	Type of service (outpatient
	hospitalization)
	Communication with doctor

with their chronic diseases. Wherever possible, the actual words of participants were later used in developing questionnaire items. For example, one of the self-efficacy questions asks, "How confident are you that you can judge when the changes in your illness mean you should visit a doctor?" This question reflects a major concern of focus group participants.

Social Psychological Theory: Self-Efficacy

The conceptual basis for the Chronic Disease Self-Management intervention and instruments was self-efficacy theory. Unlike other factors, which were open for exploration and interpretation, it was chosen at the inception of the study.

According to self-efficacy theory,

1. The strength of belief in one's capability to do a specific task or achieve a certain result is a good predictor of motivation and behavior.
2. One's self-efficacy belief can be enhanced through performance mastery, modeling, reinterpretation of symptoms, and social persuasion.

3. Enhanced self-efficacy leads to improved behavior, motivation, thinking patterns, and emotional well-being (Bandura, 1986).

Our choice of theoretical framework was based on our previous work with the Arthritis Self-Management Program. Evidence gathered from this program demonstrated that the intervention improved several aspects of participants' health behaviors and pain (Lorig, Lubeck, Kraines, Seleznick, & Holman, 1985). However, improvements in pain were not associated with changes in health behaviors (Lorig, Seleznick, et al., 1989). This surprising finding led to an exploration for the mechanisms by which the intervention altered pain. A qualitative study identified increased feelings of personal control as a key factor in changing health status (Lenker et al., 1984). Those Arthritis Self-Management program participants who experienced positive changes in pain reported increased sense of control over the symptoms of their arthritis. Those who did not experience positive changes in pain were more likely to report that there was nothing that could be done for their arthritis (Lenker et al., 1984). These feelings of personal control were operationalized as perceived self-efficacy to manage arthritis symptoms and related problems. Subsequent research demonstrated that the arthritis program had increased self-efficacy and that these changes in self-efficacy were in turn associated with improvements in pain (Lorig, Chastain, Ung, Shoor, & Holman, 1989).

In a final study of the Arthritis Self-Management program, the intervention was modified to include more efficacy-enhancing strategies. The modified arthritis program, when compared to the original program, demonstrated increased effectiveness in lowering pain and disability (Lorig & González, 1992). Because of these studies and extensive literature on the role of self-efficacy in affecting health behavior and health status, the self-efficacy construct was adopted as the central theoretical model for the Chronic Disease Self-Management Study.

Self-efficacy in dealing with chronic disease is not simply a matter of knowing what to do. Rather, it reflects a capability to organize and integrate cognitive, social, and behavioral skills to meet a variety of purposes. Coping with challenges posed by chronic disease requires not only knowledge and skills but also a belief in one's ability to use those skills in realistic contexts and a belief that the use of the skills will produce desired outcomes (Bandura, 1986).

People tend to avoid tasks and situations that they believe exceed their capabilities but readily undertake activities they judge themselves capable of performing. The Chronic Disease Self-Management Program (CDSMP) intervention uses an incremental goal setting and contracting strategy to assist in ensuring that people are successful in their efforts at change. Judgments of efficacy also determine how much effort and persistence people will expend in the face of obstacles. Those who judge themselves inefficacious in coping with the demands imposed by chronic disease(s) may dwell upon their perceived deficiencies and see difficulties as more formidable than they could be.

Knowledge of one's efficacy is derived from four sources of information: performance attainment, vicarious experiences, verbal persuasion, and physiological states (Bandura, 1986). Bandura pointed out that "performance attainment," or actual experience of the success of one's actions, is the most influential source of self-efficacy beliefs because it is based on actual skill mastery.

The success of self-efficacy approaches in health education has raised questions about some of the traditional assumptions that underlie the practice of many health education programs (Bandura, 1991; Schwarzer, 1992). Health education has often assumed that health behaviors are the only mediators of health status and that changing specific behaviors will improve health. The work of Bandura, Lorig, and others now forces us to question these assumptions in terms of the role of self-efficacy in mediating health status (Lorig & Laurin, 1985).

The Chronic Disease Self-Management Program

On the basis of the needs assessment, prior experience, literature review, and the theoretical framework of self-efficacy, CDSMP was created. This 7-week (2.5 hours per week) program is taught by pairs of trained lay leaders in community settings (senior centers, libraries, hospitals, and recreation centers). Between 10 and 15 people with chronic conditions and their significant others attend each program.

The CDSMP teaches the following content: how to develop an exercise program, cognitive symptom management, breathing exercises, problem solving, communication skills (with family, friends, and health care providers), use of medication, and dealing with the emotions of chronic illness (anger and depression).

The sessions are highly interactive, with emphasis on efficacy-enhancing strategies such as skills mastery (accomplished through weekly contracting to do specific behaviors and feedback) and modeling (accomplished by lay leaders with chronic conditions and by frequent group problem-solving sessions; Lorig, Laurent, & González, 1994).

Program Evaluation

Integrating the information from our previous intervention experience, literature review, qualitative needs assessment, previous work on outcome assessment, and theoretical orientation enabled us to identify a list of specific behavioral, self-efficacy, and outcome domains for purposes of evaluating the program. Because we had special interest in the mechanisms by which self-management programs affect health status, we chose to assess three types of self-efficacy: (a) self-efficacy for carrying out self-management behaviors, (b) self-efficacy for achieving desired health status outcomes, and (c) self-efficacy to manage the illness in general. Table 1.2 is the schematic for the final set of concepts included in the evaluation of the program.

In conclusion, this chapter has attempted to help the reader understand the overall rationale for the focus of the CDSMP. The specific measurement instruments that are described more fully in Chapter 2 were selected and developed over a 2-year period. What is important to note is that the measures, like the actual intervention, were chosen to reflect the interests and concerns of not only the investigators but also the individuals with chronic disease.

TABLE 1.2 Schematic of Concepts

Self-Management Behaviors	Self-Efficacy		Outcome Measures	
	To Perform Behaviors	To Achieve Outcomes	Health Status	Utilization
Stretching/strengthening exercise	Exercise ← regularly	Manage symptoms →	Pain and physical discomfort	Visits to physicians
Aerobic exercise			Energy/fatigue	Visits to mental health providers
Cognitive symptom management				Visits to emergency departments
Mental stress management/ relaxation		Manage shortness of breath →	Shortness of breath	Visits to other providers Hospital stays Nights in hospital Outpatient surgeries
Use of community services for tangible help				
Use of community services for emotional support	Obtain help from ← community and family/friends			
Use of community education and health support groups		Do social/recreational activities →	Activity limitation Disability	
Use of organized exercise programs		Do chores	Depressive symptoms Psychological	
Communication with physician	Communicate with ← physician	Control/manage depression →	well-being/distress Health distress	
Advance directives: Has living will/durable power of attorney		To Manage Disease in General →	Self-rated health	
Discussed with doctor				
Discussed with family				

■ References

Bandura, A. (1991). Self-efficacy mechanism and physiological activation and health promoting behavior. In V. L. Madden (Ed.), *Neurobiology of learning, emotion and affect* (pp. 229-269). New York: Raven.

Bandura, A. (1986). *Social foundations of thought and action.* Englewood Cliffs, NJ: Prentice Hall.

Basch, C. (1987). Focus group interview: An underutilized research technique for improving theory and practice in health education. *Health Education Quarterly, 14,* 411-448.

Breslow, L., & Somers, A. (1988). The periodic health examination, and updates. *Canadian Medical Association Journal, 4,* 617-626.

Butler, R. N., & Gleason, H. P. (Eds.). (1985). *Productive aging: Enhancing vitality in later life.* New York: Springer.

Clark, N. M., Becker, M. H., Janz, N. K., Lorig, K. R., Rakowski, W., & Anderson, L. (1991). Self-management of chronic disease by older adults. *Journal of Aging and Health, 3,* 3-27.

Fries, J. F. (1980). Aging, natural death and the compression of morbidity. *New England Journal of Medicine, 1,* 130-135.

Katz, S. (1983). Active life expectancy. *New England Journal of Medicine, 11,* 1218-1224.

Lenker, S. L., Lorig, K., & Gallagher, G. (1984). Reasons for the lack of association between changes in health behavior and improved health status: An explanatory study. *Patient Education and Counseling, 6*(2), 69-72.

Lorig, K. R., Chastain, R. L., Ung, E., Shoor, S., & Holman, H. R. (1989). Development and evaluation of a scale to measure perceived self-efficacy in people with arthritis. *Arthritis and Rheumatism, 32,* 37-44.

Lorig, K. R., & González, V. M. (1992). The integration of theory with practice: A 12 year case study. *Health Education Quarterly, 19,* 355-368.

Lorig, K., & Holman, H. (1993). Arthritis self-management studies: A twelve year review. *Health Education Quarterly, 20,* 17-28.

Lorig, K. R., Laurent, D. D., & González, V. M. (1994). *Chronic Disease Self-Management course leader's manual.* Palo Alto, CA: Stanford Patient Education Research Center.

Lorig, K. R., & Laurin, J. (1985). Some notions about assumptions underlying health education. *Health Education Quarterly, 12,* 231-243.

Lorig, K. R., Lubeck, D., Kraines, R. G., Seleznick, M., & Holman, H. R. (1985). Outcomes of self-help education for patients with arthritis. *Arthritis and Rheumatism, 28,* 680-685.

Lorig, K. R., Seleznick, M., Lubeck, D., Ung, E., Chastain, R. L., & Holman, H. R. (1989). The beneficial outcomes of the arthritis self-management course are not adequately explained by behavior change. *Arthritis and Rheumatism, 32,* 91-95.

Morgan, D. L. (1988). *Focus groups as qualitative research.* Newbury Park, CA: Sage.

Omenn, G. S. (1990, Summer). Prevention and the elderly: Appropriate policies. *Health Affairs, 9,* 80-93.

Rothenberg, R. B., & Koplan, J. P. (1990). Chronic disease in the 1990's. *Annual Review of Public Health, 11,* 267-296.

Rowe, J. W., & Kahn, R. L. (1987). Human aging: Usual and successful. *Science, 7,* 143-149.

Schwarzer, R. (Ed.). (1992). *Self-efficacy thought control of action.* Washington, DC: Hemisphere.

Seidel, J. V., Friese, S., & Leonard, D. C. (1995). *The ethnograph v4.0: A user's guide.* Amherst, MA: Qualis Research Associates.

U.S. Dept. of Health and Human Services. (1994). *Health, United States 1993* (DHHS Pub. No. PHS 94-1232). Hyattsville, MD: National Center for Health Statistics.

U.S. Senate Special Committee on Aging. (1988). *Aging America: Trends and projections.* Washington, DC: Government Printing Office.

Construction of Measures of Behaviors, Self-Efficacy, and Outcomes

On the basis of the conceptual framework of the self-management intervention and outcomes presented in Chapter 1, a series of self-administered measures were developed to assess each of the concepts. This chapter describes the development of those measures. It outlines the concepts, describes the methods used to select or develop measures, and provides information on the variability, reliability, and validity of the measures, using baseline data from the Chronic Disease Self-Management Program (CDSMP).

Conceptual Framework

The conceptual framework outlined in Chapter 1 was developed to organize the elements that enable a description of how well people are managing their chronic disease. These elements fall into three categories: *behaviors, beliefs about self-efficacy,* and *outcomes.* Our conceptual framework included one subcategory of behavior (self-management), three subcategories of self-efficacy beliefs (to perform specific behaviors, to manage disease generally, and to achieve outcomes), and two subcategories of outcomes (health status and health care utilization). The specific measures assessed within each of these groupings are summarized in Table 2.1. Note that many of the self-efficacy measures correspond to particular types of behavior or particular domains of health status. For example, exercise behavior and self-efficacy for exercising were both measured, as were depression and self-efficacy for managing depression.

Selection and Development of Measures ▣

Wherever possible, existing measures were selected, using the following criteria: (a) reliability and validity in the population of chronic disease patients, (b) evidence suggesting the measure's responsiveness to change in this population, and (c) brevity. Responsiveness to change is especially important as a selection criterion in intervention studies because the expected mean change is often between 0.2 and 0.4 standard deviation (Mazzuca, 1982); thus, instruments must be sensitive enough to capture this magnitude of change if it occurs. After we had selected appropriate existing measures, there were still many concepts for which new measures needed to be developed or existing measures modified.

The process of developing new measures (or modifying old ones) involved first developing an item pool (based on items from existing measures, from our experience in other self-help groups, or from comments made in focus groups), narrowing the pool down to two or three items more than we wanted in the final measure, pretesting the questionnaire on a pretest sample, and conducting multitrait scaling analyses. These are described below. On the basis of the results of the pretest scaling analyses, we revised measures as needed and developed a questionnaire for the CDSMP. Later we made minor revisions to this basic questionnaire, based on findings from several focus groups and on subsequent conceptualization of additional concepts. In addition, early in the study we determined that our initial self-efficacy scales, which were scored on a 1-to-5 Likert scale, were not detecting change. To ensure that the problem was not a lack of scale sensitivity, we changed the format to a 1-to-10 scale with labeled end points. This change in scaling appears to have improved sensitivity. Because of these changes in scaling and because new measures were added periodically throughout the study, the number of subjects on which each scale was tested varies across measures.

The final measures corresponding to the concepts outlined in Table 2.1 are presented in Table 2.2. For each measure, the table provides a definition, the number of items, the type of metric or scale, and a description of its source when applicable. All of the measures of self-management behaviors and self-efficacy (SE) were developed for this study, although some were built upon similar measures used in the arthritis self-management studies (Lorig, Chastain, Ung, Shoor, & Holman, 1989). Measures of health status were selected from the Stanford Health Assessment Questionnaire (Fries, Spitz, Kraines, & Holman, 1980; Ramey, Raynauld, & Fries, 1992) and the Medical Outcomes Study (Stewart, Sherbourne, et al., 1992).

Methods ▣

Methods of Data Collection

All data were collected via self-administered mailed questionnaires. When questionnaires were returned, they were screened for missing data. Respondents with missing data were sent a postcard asking them to call the project office between 9 a.m. and 5 p.m. and were then asked the missing questions by phone. Those who did not call within 10 days were called to recapture missing data. If questionnaires

TABLE 2.1 Overview of Measures

I. Self-Management Behaviors
 Stretching/strengthening exercise
 Aerobic exercise
 Cognitive symptom management
 Mental stress management/relaxation
 Use of community services for tangible help
 Use of community services for emotional support
 Use of community education and health support groups
 Use of organized exercise programs
 Communication with physician
 Advance directives:
   Has living will/durable power of attorney
   Discussed with doctor
   Discussed with family

II. Self-Efficacy
 Self-efficacy to perform self-management behaviors
   SE exercise regularly
   SE get information about disease
   SE obtain help from community, family, friends
   SE communicate with physician
 Self-efficacy to manage disease in general
 Self-efficacy to achieve outcomes
   SE do chores
   SE social/recreational activities
   SE manage symptoms
   SE manage shortness of breath
   SE control/manage depression

III. Outcomes
 Health status
   Disability
   Social/role activities limitations
   Pain and physical discomfort
   Energy/fatigue
   Shortness of breath
   Psychological well-being/distress
   Depressive symptoms
   Health distress
   Self-rated health
 Health care utilization
   Visits to physicians
   Visits to mental health providers
   Visits to other providers
   Visits to emergency department
   Hospital stays
   Nights in hospital
   Outpatient surgeries

---

were not returned, respondents were sent a postcard reminder after 2 weeks. After 3 weeks they were called, and after 4 weeks they received a second questionnaire. These methods resulted in return rates of over 90%.

Prior to assessment in the main study sample, 51 persons agreed to complete two questionnaires instead of one so that a test-retest study could be conducted. Subjects who agreed to take part in the test-retest reliability study received the second questionnaire 10 days after returning the first one.

Two pretests were conducted using samples of volunteers from the community who had at least one of four major chronic diseases: heart disease, lung disease, stroke, or arthritis. Volunteers were solicited through the American Heart and Lung Associations, the Arthritis Foundation, and local senior centers, community forums, and newspaper ads. There was no age limit. The first pretest sample was small and was used to test the length of the questionnaire, determine if any questions were problematic, and identify problems with item wording. The second pretest sample was larger and was used to examine item variability, item-scale correlations, and reliabilities of the draft measures. These findings were used to make revisions as needed prior to using the questionnaire in the main study.

Methods of Scale Construction

For all the self-efficacy scales and most of the health scales, we constructed and tested multi-item Likert scales using multitrait scaling (Hays & Hayashi, 1990; Stewart, Hays, & Ware, 1992b). On the remaining measures, a variety of methods of scale construction were used—for example, counting the number of behaviors performed or retaining dichotomous items (e.g., "has a living will") in their original form.

Because of the assessment of parallel self-efficacy and behavior concepts and of parallel self-efficacy and outcome concepts, one key measurement issue was the extent to which the self-efficacy measures were sufficiently unique when compared to the corresponding behaviors or outcomes. In other words, it was plausible that the amount of confidence people felt about their ability to perform a particular behavior was simply an alternative measure of their behavior. For example, reporting on one's confidence regarding the ability to walk, climb stairs, and bend without difficulty might simply be an alternative way to report on limitations in walking, climbing stairs, and bending. If this was so, the items in the self-efficacy measure and the corresponding health outcome measure would be highly correlated. Multitrait scaling analysis was used to address this problem.

A particular strength of multitrait scaling analysis for developing our Likert scales of self-efficacy was that it allowed tests of whether items in the hypothesized efficacy scales were too highly related to the parallel behavior or outcome scales. Another strength of multitrait scaling was that it is a confirmatory approach that tests the adequacy of a hypothesized scale structure. Thus, it is especially appropriate for testing measures for which there is a strong theoretical basis and a history of measurement.

Multitrait scaling analysis is based on the traditional Likert (1932) method of summated ratings. Five steps were followed (Stewart, Hays, & Ware, 1992b) to determine whether

1. Each item in the hypothesized scale correlated substantially with the sum of the other items in the scale (item-convergence criterion); a fairly stringent standard of 0.40 was used;

TABLE 2.2 Definition of Measures

Measure	No. of Items	Metric/Type of Scale	Source
Self-Management Behaviors			
Stretching/strengthening exercise: Time in past week spent doing stretching/strengthening exercises	1	Single-item; ordinal scale converted into minutes spent	New measure
Aerobic exercise: Time in past week spent doing walking for exercise, swimming or aquatic exercise, bicycling or stationary bike, aerobic exercise equipment, other aerobic exercise	5	Sum of ordinal scales converted to minutes spent	New measure
Cognitive symptom management: When feeling bad or having pain or symptoms, frequency of trying various cognitive strategies (e.g., trying to feel distant from the discomfort, talking to self in positive ways, practicing visualization)	6	Likert scale	New measure
Mental stress management/relaxation: Number of times in past week did mental stress management or cognitive relaxation techniques (technique verified by asking what they did; 1 = *none*, 2 = *1-7 times per week or up to daily*, 3 = *8 or more times per week*)	1	Number of times categorized into ordinal scale with three categories	New measure
Use of community services for tangible help: Received help in past 6 months from other than family/friends for housecleaning, yardwork, home maintenance, meals, errands, personal hygiene, transportation	7	Count of resources	New measure
Use of community services for emotional support: Received emotional support/ counseling in past 6 months from other than family/friends	1	Dichotomous item	New measure
Use of community education and health support groups—hours: Total hours spent in classes/lectures/support groups about health problem in past 6 months outside of this study	1	Hours attended	New measure
Use of organized exercise programs—hours: Total hours spent in organized exercise programs (such as walking clubs, aerobic classes, water exercise) in past 6 months	1	Hours attended	New measure
Communication with physician: When visiting physician, frequency of preparing list of questions, asking questions about things one doesn't know/understand, discussing personal problems related to illness	3	Likert scale	New measure
Advance directives: Has living will/durable power of attorney	1	Dichotomous item	New measure
Discussed wishes with doctor in event of serious illness or impending death	1	Dichotomous item	New measure
Discussed wishes with family in event of serious illness or impending death	1	Dichotomous item	New measure

TABLE 2.2 *Continued*

Measure	No. of Items	Metric/Type of Scale	Source
Self-Efficacy to Perform Self-Management Behaviors			
SE exercise regularly: Confidence that one can do flexibility/strengthening exercises 3-4 times weekly, do aerobic exercises 3-4 times weekly, exercise without making symptoms worse	3	Likert scale	New measure
SE get information about disease: Confidence that one can get information about disease from community resources	1	Likert scale	New measure
SE obtain help from community, family, friends: Confidence that one can get emotional support and help with daily tasks from community resources and from family and friends	4	Likert scale	New measure
SE communicate with physician: Confidence that one can ask doctor about things of concern, discuss openly any personal problems related to illness, work out differences if any arise	3	Likert scale	New measure
Self-Efficacy to Manage Disease in General			
SE manage disease in general: Confidence that one can manage condition on regular basis, judge when changes mean should visit a doctor, do tasks needed to manage condition so as to reduce need to see doctor, reduce emotional distress caused by condition, and do things other than take medications to reduce effect of illness on everyday life	5	Likert scale	New measure
Self-Efficacy to Achieve Outcomes			
SE do chores: Confidence that one can complete household chores, get errands done, get shopping done despite health problems	3	Likert scale	New measure
SE social/recreational activities: Confidence that one can continue hobbies/recreation, continue to do things liked socially	2	Likert scale	New measure
SE manage symptoms: Confidence that one can reduce pain, keep fatigue and pain from interfering, keep other symptoms from interfering, control symptoms so they don't interfere with things	4	Likert scale	New measure
SE manage shortness of breath: Confidence that one can keep shortness of breath from interfering	1	Single-item scale	New measure
SE control/manage depression: Confidence that one can keep from feeling sad, discouraged, lonely and can do something to feel better when feeling sad, discouraged, lonely	6	Likert scale	New measure
Health Status			
Disability: Difficulty in past 4 weeks with dressing and grooming, arising, eating, walking, hygiene, reaching, gripping, and activities	22	Likert scale of 8 categories of items	Stanford Health Assessment Questionnaire, disability scale, modified (Fries et al., 1980; Ramey et al., 1992). See Appendix C for modifications.

continued

TABLE 2.2 *Continued*

Measure	No. of Items	Metric/Type of Scale	Source
Social/role activities limitations: Extent to which health has interfered with social and recreational activities, chores, errands, and shopping over the past 4 weeks	4	Likert scale	New measure
Pain and physical discomfort (scale): Pain and physical discomfort intensity, frequency, duration over past 4 weeks	5	Likert scale	MOS pain severity modified to omit skip pattern and to add "physical discomfort" to item stems (Sherbourne, 1992)
Pain and physical discomfort (item): Rating of physical discomfort or pain on a visual analogue scale from no pain to pain as bad as it could be	1	Visual analogue	
Energy/fatigue: Amount of time in past 4 weeks that one felt full of pep, energetic, worn out, tired, had enough energy to do the things one wanted to do	5	Likert scale	MOS energy/fatigue (Stewart, Hays, & Ware, 1992a)
Shortness of breath: Extent to which one was troubled by shortness of breath when doing normal activities over past 4 weeks	1	Ordinal item	New measure
Psychological well-being/distress: Summary index of depression, anxiety, positive affect. Amount of time in past 4 weeks that one was a very nervous person, downhearted, down in the dumps, happy person, calm and peaceful	5	Likert scale	MOS Mental Health Index I (Stewart, Hays, & Ware, 1988; Ware, Sherbourne, & Davies, 1992; Ware & Sherbourne, 1992)
Depressive symptoms MOS: Amount of time in past 4 weeks that one felt in low spirits, downhearted, depressed, nothing to look forward to, not in firm control of behavior, not emotionally stable	8	Likert scale	MOS Depression/ Behavioral-Emotional Control Index I (Stewart, Ware, Sherbourne, & Wells, 1992)
Depressive symptoms CES-D: Depressive symptoms over past week	20	Likert scale	Radloff, 1977
Health distress: Amount of time in past 4 weeks that one felt distressed about health (e.g., discouraged, worried, fearful, frustrated by health problems)	4	Likert scale	MOS health distress modified slightly (Stewart, Hays, & Ware, 1992a, 4 of 6 items); "afraid because of your health" changed to "fearful about future health"; "frustrated about your health" changed to "frustrated by your health problems"
Self-rated health: Rating of health as excellent, very good, good, fair, or poor	1	Single-item scale	National Center for Health Statistics, 1991; Ware, Nelson, Sherbourne, & Stewart, 1992
Health Care Utilization in Past 6 Months			
Visits to physicians: Number of visits to a physician other than a psychiatrist in past 6 months	1	Count of visits	Standard
Visits to mental health providers: Number of visits to psychiatrists, psychologists, or other mental health counselors in past 6 months	2	Count of visits	New measure

TABLE 2.2 *Continued*

Measure	No. of Items	Metric/Type of Scale	Source
Visits to emergency department: Number of visits to emergency room in past 6 months	1	Count of visits	Standard
Visits to other providers: Number of visits to nurse practitioner, physician's assistant, home health nurse, physical/occupational or respiratory therapist in past 6 months	3	Count of visits	New measure
Number of hospital stays: Number of times that one stayed in hospital overnight or longer in past 6 months	1	Count of stays	Standard
Nights in hospital: Number of total nights that one stayed in hospital overnight in past 6 months; those with no stays are assigned a zero	1	Count of nights	Standard
Outpatient surgeries: Number of times in past 6 months that one had outpatient surgery (did not stay overnight in hospital)	1	Count of times	New measure

2. Each item correlated significantly more highly with the construct it was hypothesized to measure than with other constructs (item-discrimination criterion); this criterion was met if the correlation between the item and its hypothesized scale was greater than or equal to two standard errors of the correlation. In our analyses, one standard error equaled about .05;

3. Items in the same scale contained the same proportion of information about the construct (tested for approximately equal item-scale correlations);

4. Items measuring the same construct had equal variances and therefore did not need to be standardized before being combined into the same scale.

If items in the hypothesized groupings satisfied these criteria, simple summation of items (or averaging of nonmissing items) to construct the scale was appropriate. To accomplish these tests, a matrix of item-scale correlations was examined in which each row represented one of the items and each column represented the various scales being tested. Each row consisted of the item-scale correlation. For scales in which the item was hypothesized to be included, the item-scale correlation was corrected for overlap: that is, the correlation was that between the item and the sum of the remaining items. These analyses were performed using the Multitrait Analysis Program.[1]

For purposes of scale testing, persons with missing data were omitted from the analysis. Once the final scales were determined, for purposes of calculating derived scores, we estimated scores for those with any missing data on items within a scale by calculating the score based on the remaining items. Persons missing more than one quarter of the items in a scale were assigned a missing scale value.

Because of the large number of measures being tested and the need to evaluate each efficacy scale in relation to its corresponding behavioral or outcome measure, we conducted a series of multitrait scaling analyses. Each of these analyses included a particular subset of scales, as follows: (a) behaviors only, (b) efficacy scales only, (c) health scales only, (d) efficacy for achieving outcomes with the actual outcomes, and (e) efficacy for performing various behaviors with the actual behaviors. This enabled us to develop scales within each set that were distinct: that is, scales in which items did not correlate more highly with any other scale than the scale in which the item was hypothesized to belong.

Variability

Variability pertains to the extent to which each measure has a full range of scale values represented and is approximately normally distributed. We examined each final measure for variability, noting whether all scale levels were represented and whether there were potential floor or ceiling effects (a large proportion of the sample scoring at the highest or lowest end of the measure). To the extent that scores were variable and somewhat normally distributed, changes in either the positive or negative direction were more likely to be detected.

Reliability

Reliability pertains to the consistency of the score or the extent to which scores are free of random error. Reliability coefficients are estimates of the proportion of total variance that is true score variance as opposed to error variance. Reliability for multi-item scales was tested using internal-consistency and test-retest methods. For single-item measures and for those derived as simple counts, we depended solely on test-retest methods. Ten-day test-retest reliability was examined in a subsample of individuals enrolled as comparison controls somewhat early in the study. Hence, test-retest reliability was not available on single-item measures added later. This time period was selected as one in which these concepts could be considered relatively stable and one that was long enough so that participants would not mind completing the questionnaires again. Although some have suggested that reliabilities above .50 are acceptable for group comparisons (Nunnally, 1978), our goal was to achieve reliability coefficients above .70 (Stewart, Hays, & Ware, 1992b).

Validity

Validity refers to the extent to which a score measures what it is intended to measure and does not measure what it is not intended to measure. Validating a measure or set of measures is a process of accumulating many different kinds of evidence to learn about the meaning of a score or of differences or changes in scores. Studies of the validity of health and health-related measures depend primarily on construct validity methods (Stewart, Hays, & Ware, 1992c).

In addition to the item convergent and discriminant validity tests conducted as part of the multitrait scaling analyses (described above), construct validity of all of the resulting scales was examined by evaluating correlations among the various measures to determine whether correlations corresponded to hypotheses and to ensure that they were low enough to indicate that the measures were independent. We examined correlations among the self-management behavior measures, among the self-efficacy measures, among the health status measures, and among the health care utilization measures. For the self-efficacy measures, we also evaluated the correlations between each measure and its corresponding behavior or outcome measure to ensure that the self-efficacy measure was not highly correlated with the corresponding measure. In addition, we included other related measures to examine the extent to which efficacy measures were correlated with similar measures. To some extent, these studies of the validity of the self-efficacy measures were a confirmation of the item discriminant validity analyses during the multitrait scaling. We also examined the extent to which intercorrelations among the health measures were similar to those in other studies. We primarily compared the pattern of correlations with those obtained in the Medical Outcomes Study (MOS), a study of chronically ill individuals (Stewart, Sherbourne, et al., 1992). The MOS sample consisted of 3,053 adults aged 18 to 98 (mean age = 54) who were 61% female and 79% white and had an average education of 13 years. MOS patients had one or more chronic conditions, including hypertension, diabetes, congestive heart failure, recent myocardial infarction, major depression, and/or depressive symptoms. Thus, the two samples were somewhat comparable, except that the chronic disease self-management sample consisted of individuals who had also sought out a self-management course (and would thus be expected to be somewhat more ill than the MOS patients).

Self-reports of utilization of health care were validated through the use of chart audits on a subset of 36 subjects enrolled at one health maintenance organization. These subjects were selected for this study to minimize the possibility that they would have multiple medical records. All visits occurring within the 6-month period prior to the self-reported utilization were abstracted. Prior to this abstraction, inter-rater reliability was examined by having two investigators independently abstract data from seven charts. The two abstractors were 100% in accord for data on six of the charts and 93% in accord for the seventh chart. Because of this high rate of inter-rater reliability, the final 29 charts were abstracted by only one investigator. All charts were abstracted twice by the same investigator at two different times. Any difficulties in reading or understanding the information in the charts were resolved by a physician working in the facility, who also served as the second abstractor for the first seven charts. Visits were classified into the following measures: number of outpatient visits to physicians, number of emergency department visits, number of hospitalizations, and number of nights in the hospital. Urgent care visits were classified along with emergency department visits. The number of visits in the chart was compared to the number based on self-reports, and any discrepancy was considered a reporting error. In addition, the discrepancy was also calculated as a proportion of the actual visits made. For example, if a person reported only one of two visits, the proportional error was 50%. However, if a person reported 9 of 10 visits, the proportional error was 10%.

Results

Sample

The measurement analyses reported here were conducted on the baseline questionnaire from 1,130 individuals enrolled in the self-management courses or enrolled in the comparison-control group. Sample characteristics are described in Table 2.3.

TABLE 2.3 Sample Characteristics ($N = 1,130$)

Age (years)	
Range	39.2-90.5
Mean (standard deviation)	64.4 (10.9)
Education (years)	
Range	6-23
Mean (standard deviation)	14.8 (2.9)
Gender (%)	
Female	68
Male	32
Marital status (%)	
Married	56.5
Single	9.2
Separated	1.5
Divorced	16.0
Widowed	16.8
Ethnicity (%)	
White (Non-Hispanic)	91.1
Black (Non-Hispanic)	1.8
Hispanic	3.7
Asian/Pacific Islander	1.9
Filipino	0.5
American Indian	0.2
Other	0.7
Self-rated health (%)	
Excellent	3.1
Very good	14.0
Good	41.9
Fair	32.9
Poor	8.1

As shown there, the sample included a broad age range (mean age = 64.4) and was 68% female, mostly white, and well educated (mean years of education = 14.8). Only 3% rated their health as excellent. The pretest sample ($N = 51$) did not differ from the larger sample in any significant way.

All subjects who had completed questionnaire data on health care utilization and were enrolled from a specific HMO clinic (36 people) were selected for a study to compare self-reported utilization with that recorded in their charts. The demographics of this group (the chart audit sample) differed only slightly from the total sample (mean age = 64.3 years, 75% female, mean education = 13.5 years). The average number of chronic conditions in this group was 2.3. Charts were reviewed to assess utilization during the 6-month period corresponding to that reported in the questionnaire.

Scale Construction

Behaviors

We conducted multitrait analyses on the two multi-item behavioral constructs: cognitive symptom management and communication with physician. All items in these scales met criteria of item convergence and item discrimination: that is, they correlated at least .40 with the sum of other items in the scale and correlated significantly more highly with the hypothesized scale than with the other scale in the matrix.

For many of the remaining behavior scales, we used simple counts of various behaviors (e.g., a count of the number of community resources used over some specified time period). For several items, respondents were asked to report the number of hours or the number of days they had attended certain classes (e.g., exercise classes, health education classes). Because these types of data tend to be skewed, with the majority of individuals reporting no hours or days and a long tail of individuals reporting high numbers of hours or days, we created an ordinal transformation of each scale *in addition to* the original raw score. The ordinal levels were designed to correspond to meaningful categories of the numbers reported, as well as to achieve roughly equivalent proportions of individuals in the nonzero categories. For the two continuous scales that were transformed (use of community education services and use of organized exercise programs), we provide scoring rules on both the original data (hours) and the transformed data (categories) in Appendix A. Readers can then code these scales as they wish. In our study, preliminary analyses suggested that the two methods of scoring were comparable in terms of correlations with other measures. However, for smaller studies, the ordinal transformations should provide scores with better distributions because outliers are more critical in small samples.

Self-Efficacy

All items in the final self-efficacy scales met criteria of item convergence: That is, all item-scale correlations (corrected for overlap) exceeded .50, which was well above our stringent minimum of .40. Nearly all items correlated significantly more highly with their own scale than with any other self-efficacy scale. A few items were "probable errors"—that is, correlated within two standard errors of another scale. However, in all cases, the items were correlating at least one standard error higher with their own scale, and the errors tended to be randomly distributed across the various items. Thus, we concluded that the final scales were satisfactory.

Outcomes

Health Status. For the multi-item health scales (excluding the CES-D scale), all item-scale correlations were above .40, thus meeting the item-convergence criterion. All items also met our stringent item-discrimination criterion: that is, they correlated at least two standard errors higher with their hypothesized scale than with any other scale. When the CES-D scale was included in the matrix instead of the MOS depression scale, the sample size dropped ($N = 237$) because this scale was added later in the study. Item-scale correlations for the CES-D ranged from .31 to .70, and 6 of the 20 items correlated less than .40 with the total scale score (corrected for overlap). This suggests that this scale consists of items that are quite heterogeneous. Further, there were a number of probable scaling errors associated with items in the CES-D. Most of the errors consisted of items correlating within two standard errors (sometimes higher, sometimes lower than the correlation with the CES-D scale) with the health distress, energy/fatigue, and pain and physical discomfort scales. For example, the item *felt fearful* correlated more highly with the health distress scale, and the *everything was an effort* item correlated equally with the energy/fatigue and social/role activities limitations scales. These results suggest that this scale, which includes a number of somatic items in addition to depressed affect items, may be confounded with physical problems in samples of chronically ill persons. We did not include the CES-D and MOS depression scales in the same multitrait scaling matrix because our intention was to test these as alternative approaches to assessing depression.

Health Care Utilization. Utilization measures were scored primarily in terms of the metric in which they were asked (e.g., number of visits to physicians). Thus, no scaling studies per se were required for scale construction.

Descriptive Statistics, Reliability Coefficients

In Table 2.4, the baseline characteristics of each measure are presented, including the number of items, sample size (N), mean, standard deviation (SD), possible range, observed range, internal consistency (IC) and test-retest (TR) reliability coefficient(s), and range of item-scale correlations for multi-item Likert scales. The test-retest coefficients were based on the test-retest sample described earlier. As noted earlier, some scales were added after the beginning of the study; this accounts for differences in sample size in the various scales.

Behaviors

Most self-management behavior measures were slightly skewed, with the majority of respondents scoring at the lower end (not performing each behavior). Because the intervention was designed to increase these behaviors, this was not viewed as a problem for this study. Only one measure was skewed in the positive direction, the advance directives measure pertaining to discussing one's wishes with one's family: 70% reported having discussed their wishes with their families.

The range of test-retest reliability coefficients was .56 to .92, and the range of internal-consistency coefficients was .70 to .75. Four measures had reliabilities lower than our standard of .70: stretching/strengthening exercise ($r = .56$), mental stress management/relaxation ($r = .66$), use of organized exercise classes ($r = .55$), and use of community services for educational support ($r = .59$). Thus, the reliability of these scales could be improved.

Self-Efficacy

Most of the self-efficacy measures tended to have means slightly above the midpoint of the 10-point scale (from 1 to 2 points above). Thus, the scales were reasonably well distributed, although slightly skewed, with subjects tending to report high efficacy. The highest means were 7.37 for self-efficacy to get information on their disease and 7.30 for self-efficacy to communicate with physicians. The lowest self-efficacy means were for managing symptoms of the disease (5.88) and managing shortness of breath (5.87). Thus, no floor or ceiling effects were observed.

Test-retest reliability coefficients ranged from .82 to .89, and internal-consistency coefficients from .77 to .92. Thus, the reliability of all of the self-efficacy scales was quite good.

Outcomes

Health Status. The nature of the distributions of the health status scales varied across scales. The mean disability score was .84, which is within one standard deviation of a perfect score. This suggests possible ceiling effects, which might make it difficult to observe improvement in this measure in this sample. This score is comparable to the disability reported by a community sample of people with arthritis who completed an arthritis self-management course (Lorig, Lubeck, Kraines, Seleznick, & Holman, 1985). The social/role activities limitations scale was slightly skewed, with most individuals having fewer limitations, but there did not appear to be such ceiling effects in this measure. Both of the pain and physical discomfort scales were well distributed, with the mean roughly near the midpoint of the scales. The energy/fatigue scale was also roughly normally distributed, although the skew was such that people tended to have fatigue. The energy/ fatigue score was about one half of a standard deviation lower than that observed in the MOS chronically ill patients. The shortness-of-breath scale was slightly skewed with most individuals not having shortness of breath.

The psychological well-being/distress measure was also roughly normally distributed, with mean scores slightly above the midpoint. This mean score (when transformed to correspond to the MOS method of scoring) was nearly identical to that observed in the MOS sample of chronically ill patients (including some with depression; Stewart, Ware, Sherbourne, & Wells, 1992). The mean score on the MOS depressive symptoms scale was slightly skewed toward fewer people having depressive symptoms. However, this mean is about one third of a standard deviation higher (more depressed) than the mean in the MOS sample, which included a number of patients with depression. The mean CES-D score was 16.72, which is considerably higher (more depressed) than that for a general population sample of community residents (mean ranging from 7.5 to 12.7; Devins & Orme, 1985). The mean CES-D score for people enrolled in an arthritis self-management course was 12 to 13. Thus, our results indicate that this sample had considerable depressive symptoms. Although the two depressive symptoms measures allow for substantial improvement on depressive symptoms, the relative distributions suggest that this sample had more depressive symptoms than other chronic disease samples. It is possible that disease symptoms such as fatigue (which was high in this sample) confounded the depression scores and artificially increased them, as was suggested by the item-scale correlation studies described above. Indeed, Blalock and her colleagues examined this issue in patients with rheumatoid arthritis; although some items were apparently affected by the disease process, they concluded that the magnitude of the bias was sufficiently small that the measure could be used without affecting study findings (Blalock, DeVellis, Brown, & Wallston, 1989).

The self-rated health and health distress measures were normally distributed, with mean scores lying roughly midway between the end points. However, the health distress score was one standard deviation higher than that observed in the MOS

TABLE 2.4 Baseline Characteristics of Measures

Measure[a]	No. of Items	N	Mean	SD	Possible Range	Observed Range	IC Reliability[b]	TR Reliability[c]	Range of Item-Scale Correlations
Self-Management Behaviors									
Stretching/strengthening exercise (minutes/week)	1	1,127	40.1	54.8	—	0-180	—	.56	—
Aerobic exercise (minutes/week)	5	1,130	90.6	90.9	—	0-540	—	.72	—
Cognitive symptom management	6	1,129	1.33	0.91	0-5	0-4.83	.75	.83	.36-.58
Mental stress management/ relaxation	1	1,129	1.28	0.53	1-3	1-3	—	.66	—
Use of community services:									
For tangible help	7	1,129	1.44	1.58	0-7	0-7	.70	.79	—
For emotional support	1	1,128	0.18	0.38	0-1	0-1	—	.59	—
Use of community education and health support groups:									
Classes/lectures/support groups (hours last 6 months)	1	237	1.73	4.69	—	0-33	—	—	—
Use of organized exercise programs (hours/last 6 months)	1	1,129	8.40	27.14	—	0-250	—	.72	—
Communication with physician	3	1,130	3.08	1.20	0-5	0-5	.73	.89	.49-.66
Advance directives:									
Has living will, durable power of attorney	1	1,127	0.48	0.50	0-1	0-1	—	.92	—
Discussed with doctor	1	891	0.22	0.41	0-1	0-1	—	.74	—
Discussed with family	1	891	0.70	0.46	0-1	0-1	—	.83	—
Self-Efficacy to Perform Self-Management Behaviors									
SE exercise regularly	3	478	6.30	2.70	1-10	1-10	.83	.86	.68-.71
SE get information on disease	1	478	7.37	2.65	1-10	1-10	—	.72	—
SE obtain help from community, family, friends	4	478	6.18	2.42	1-10	1-10	.77	.85	.55-.64
SE communicate with physician	3	477	7.30	2.71	1-10	1-10	.90	.88	.80-.83
General Self-Efficacy									
SE manage disease in general	5	292	6.92	2.15	1-10	1-10	.87	—	.58-.79
Self-Efficacy to Achieve Outcomes									
SE do chores	3	478	6.29	2.70	1-10	1-10	.91	.86	.72-.90
SE do social/recreational activities	2	478	6.50	2.65	1-10	1-10	.82	.84	.70
SE manage symptoms	4	478	5.88	2.40	1-10	1-10	.91	.89	.66-.86
SE manage shortness of breath[d]	1	280	5.87	2.97	1-10	1-10	—	.82	—
SE control/manage depression	6	478	6.51	2.23	1-10	1-10	.92	.82	.74-.82
Health Status									
Disability (–)	8	1,130	.84	.62	0-3	0-3	.86	.95	.42-.72
Social/role activities limitations (–)	4	1,130	1.70	1.11	0-4	0-4	.91	.68	.77-.80
Pain and physical discomfort scale (–)	5	1,130	60.0	22.2	0-100	0-100	.88	.91	.61-.79
Pain and physical discomfort item (–)	1	237	4.50	2.62	0-10	0-10	—	.79[e]	—

TABLE 2.4 *Continued*

Measure[a]	No. of Items	N	Mean	SD	Possible Range	Observed Range	IC Reliability[b]	TR Reliability[c]	Range of Item-Scale Correlations
Energy/fatigue	5	1,130	2.16	1.08	0-5	0-5	.89	.85	.68-.76
Shortness of breath (–)	1	1,129	1.53	1.31	0-4	0-4	—	.87	—
Psychological well-being/distress	5	1,130	3.43	0.90	0-5	0-5	.83	.82	—
Depressive symptoms MOS (–)	8	1,130	1.33	.90	0-5	0-4.38	.90	.82	.52-.83
Depressive symptoms CES-D (–)	20	239	16.72	9.56	0-60	1-47	.87	—	.31-.71
Self-rated health (–)	1	1,129	3.29	.91	1-5	1-5	—	.92	—
Health distress	4	1,130	2.04	1.16	0-5	0-5	.87	.87	.67-.75
Health Care Utilization in Past 6 Months									
Visits to physicians	1	1,128	5.33	5.23	—	0-54	—	.76	—
Visits to mental health providers	2	1,129	0.86	3.70	—	0-42	—	.82	—
Visits to emergency department	1	1,129	0.40	.93	—	0-9	—	.94	—
Visits to other providers	3	1,130	2.32	7.26	—	0-104	—	.84	—
Hospital stays	1	1,129	0.23	0.76	—	0-14	—	.89	—
Nights in hospital	1	1,130	1.31	5.53	—	0-116	—	.97	—
Outpatient surgeries	1	1,129	0.16	0.57	—	0-12	—	.45	—

a. High score indicates better health, greater efficacy, except where indicated with (–).
b. Internal-consistency (IC) reliability.
c. 10-day test-retest (TR) reliability, subset of sample (*N* = 51).
d. Only measured on those who reported having shortness of breath.
e. Alternate forms reliability.

sample, suggesting substantially more distress in the chronic disease self-management sample.

Health Care Utilization. Utilization scores over the prior 6 months were reasonable for this group of chronically ill persons. For example, people 65 years of age and above had 9.3 to 12.8 physician visits in 1993 (U.S. Dept. of Health and Human Services, 1995).

Validity

Behaviors

Correlations among the self-management behaviors are shown in Table 2.5. The absolute magnitude of the correlations ranged from .00 to .39, with the largest correlation (.39) between cognitive symptom management and mental stress management/relaxation. The next highest correlation was between the two exercise measures (aerobic exercise and stretching/strengthening). These findings suggest that these self-management behaviors are considerably independent of one another and that consequently all could be included in one study without concern for overlap.

Self-Efficacy

Correlations among the self-efficacy measures are shown in Table 2.6, with internal-consistency reliabilities on the diagonal. Correlations among the specific

TABLE 2.5 Correlations Among Self-Management Behaviors ($N = 1,130$)

		SS	AE	CS	MS	TN	EM	CL	EX	MD
Stretching/strengthening exercise	SS	(.56)								
Aerobic exercise	AE	.29	(.72)							
Cognitive symptom management	CS	.18	.14	(.83)						
Mental stress management/ relaxation	MS	.16	.06	.39	(.66)					
Use of community services for tangible help	TN	.04	−.06	.09	.04	(.79)				
Use of community services for emotional support	EM	.03	.02	.10	.16	.22	(.59)			
Classes/lectures/support groups—hours	CL	.14	.02	.16	.12	.02	.18	(NA)		
Use of organized exercise programs—hours	EX	.26	.16	.03	.02	.07	.06	.17	(.72)	
Communication with physician	MD	.08	.04	.17	.11	.00	.02	.05	.04	(.89)

NOTE: Reliability estimates are on the diagonal.

measures (excluding the overall management of disease index) ranged from .14 to .68. The largest correlations were between self-efficacy for managing symptoms and self-efficacy for continuing one's social and recreational activities ($r = .67$) and between managing symptoms and managing depression ($r = .68$). The correlations between the general self-efficacy to manage disease index and the specific scales ranged from .36 to .77 (median = .55). Because the index to manage disease in general was intended to be a summary index, we expected these correlations to be high. If we examine the pattern of correlations, it appears that this summary index more closely taps efficacy for managing symptoms (depression, pain, fatigue) and for obtaining help.

Outcomes

Health Status. Correlations among the health status measures are shown in Table 2.7. It should be noted that this matrix of correlations is among all measures, including several that overlap conceptually or in terms of actual items. Thus, this table is descriptive only and is not intended to demonstrate independence among all 11 measures. The absolute magnitude of the correlations ranged from .14 to .90. The largest correlation of .90 was between depression and the psychological well-being/distress index (which contained two of the depression items). Thus, this correlation was expected to be high. The next highest correlation was between health distress and depressive symptoms ($r = .61$) and between health distress and psychological well-being/distress ($r = -.60$). The self-rated health item had the most even pattern of correlations (ranging from .28 to .46 absolute magnitude), as would be expected given the general nature of this measure.

TABLE 2.6 Correlations Among Self-Efficacy Measures (*N* = 292-478)

		EX	*IN*	*FF*	*MD*	*CH*	*SR*	*SX*	*SB*	*DP*	*DS*
Specific Measures											
SE exercise regularly	EX	(.86)									
SE get information	IN	.26	(.72)								
SE obtain help from community, family, friends	FF	.30	.43	(.77)							
SE communicate with physician	MD	.31	.33	.39	(.90)						
SE do chores	CH	.58	.17	.29	.24	(.91)					
SE social/ recreational activities	SR	.50	.30	.50	.33	.63	(.82)				
SE manage symptoms	SX	.39	.40	.59	.32	.52	.63	(.90)			
SE manage shortness of breath	SB	.37	.27	.35	.14	.40	.48	.62	(.82)		
SE control/ manage depression	DP	.29	.46	.63	.32	.32	.55	.68	.38	(.92)	
General Summary Index											
SE manage disease	DS	.36	.53	.60	.43	.37	.60	.77	.56	.70	(.87)

NOTE: Reliability estimates are on the diagonal.

For the MOS scales, we compared these correlations to those obtained in the MOS sample of chronically ill patients (Stewart, Sherbourne, et al., 1992). Correlations between the pain index and all other measures tended to be slightly higher in the MOS sample than in this sample, perhaps due to the modification in this study to include physical discomfort in addition to pain. For those scales taken from the MOS and for those scales that were similar to MOS measures (e.g., the disability scale, which is somewhat similar in item content to the MOS physical functioning scale), we compared scale-scale correlations with those obtained for identical or similar scales in the MOS sample of chronically ill patients. Correlations were remarkably similar, despite the various modifications made to some of the MOS scales. For example, the disability scale correlated .46 with the pain severity scale, and in the MOS, physical functioning correlated .48 with the pain severity scale. Similarly, energy/fatigue correlated −.49 with the depressive symptoms scale, whereas in the MOS the correlation between these two scales was −.52. Correlations between health distress and depressive symptoms and between health distress and psychological well-being/distress were virtually identical in the two samples.

TABLE 2.7 Correlations Among Health Status Measures (N = 1,130)

		DIS	SOC	PNS	PNI	ENF	SOB	DEP	CES	PSY	HDS	SRH
Disability (–)	DIS	(.94)										
Social/role activities limitations (–)	SOC	.58	(.90)									
Pain and physical discomfort scale (–)	PNS	.46	.49	(.89)								
Pain and physical discomfort item (–)	PNI	.45	.58	.85	(.79)							
Energy/fatigue	ENF	–.43	–.58	–.38	–.44	(.91)						
Shortness of breath (–)	SOB	.16	.29	.14	.14	–.35	(.85)					
Depressive symptoms MOS (–)	DEP	.21	.38	.25	.35	–.49	.18	(.90)				
Depressive symptoms CES-D	CES	.26	.43	.33	.34	–.45	.16	.74	(.87)			
Psychological well-being/distress	PSY	–.21	–.38	–.26	–.37	.50	–.19	–.90[a]	–.72	(.83)		
Health distress (–)	HDS	.30	.52	.38	.36	–.52	.25	.61	.63	–.60	(.86)	
Self-rated health (–)	SRH	.34	.44	.28	.41	–.46	.42	.29	.36	–.30	.37	(.92)

NOTE: A (–) means that higher score indicates poorer health. Reliability estimates are on the diagonal. All coefficients are significant (p < .001).
a. High coefficient due to overlapping items.

Health Care Utilization. Correlations among the utilization measures are shown in Table 2.8. These correlations ranged from .00 to .60, with the highest correlation between the number of hospital stays and the number of nights in the hospital, as would be expected. Mental health visits were the least correlated with other measures, ranging from .00 to .09.

Self-Efficacy and Corresponding Measures

Correlations between self-efficacy scales and the corresponding behaviors or outcomes are shown in Table 2.9. The absolute magnitude of the correlations between self-management behaviors and self-efficacy to perform the behaviors ranged from .01 to .41. The highest correlation was between self-efficacy for communicating with the physician and actual communication with the physician (r = .41). Multitrait scaling studies of the four multi-item scales pertaining to behaviors and the corresponding self-efficacy for performing those behaviors confirmed that the self-efficacy and the behavior scales were measuring different constructs. We are thus reassured that the scales measuring self-efficacy to perform behaviors are sufficiently independent of the actual behaviors that they can be interpreted as distinct scales.

The absolute magnitude of the correlations between the health outcomes and self-efficacy to achieve those outcomes ranged from .14 to .75. The largest correlation (and the cause for greatest concern) is between self-efficacy for managing depression and three of the psychological scales: depressive symptoms (–.75), CES-D depression (–.68), and psychological well-being/distress (.72). However, on examination of the multitrait scaling analysis in which these were included together, items in these scales were discriminating sufficiently well for us to feel confident

TABLE 2.8 Correlations Among Health Care Utilization Measures ($N = 1,130$)

		MD	MH	ER	OP	HS	HN	OP
Visits to physicians	MD	(.76)						
Visits to mental health providers	MH	.09	(.82)					
Visits to emergency department	ER	.28	.06	(.94)				
Visits to other providers	OP	.17	.08	.10	(.84)			
Hospital stays	HS	.22	.01	.40	.13	(.89)		
Nights in hospital	HN	.15	.00	.37	.16	.60	(.97)	
Outpatient surgeries	OP	.18	.03	.10	.03	.03	.03	(.45)

NOTE: Reliability estimates are on the diagonal.

that they could be used as distinct measures. The remaining correlations were of less concern, falling below .65.

Health Care Utilization Versus Chart Reviews

In the analysis of chart reviews, the total number of self-reported visits to physicians over the past 6 months ranged from 1 to 15, and the range of visits recorded in the charts was from 1 to 16. The total number of visits reported was 151, and the total number found in the charts was 183, resulting in a 17% underreporting of visits. Thirty-six percent of subjects accurately reported the number of outpatient visits, 19% underreported, and 44% overreported. The average number of visits underreported was 2.7, and the average number of visits overreported was 1.6. Thus, there was a tendency toward underreporting in the total sample, and those who underreported made greater errors on average. Underreporters tended to be those with more actual visits during the 6-month period. It should be noted that although individuals' self-report of utilization is somewhat unreliable, the group report is much more reliable. Because most intervention studies look at change, self-report should be reliable, especially if the change across individuals is reported as a percentage of initial levels instead of in absolute numbers. This is because there is no need to believe that reporting errors will differ from one time period to the next.

In this data set, there were few emergency visits and hospitalizations reported—16 emergency department visits and eight hospitalizations. Thus, the percentage of subjects who accurately reported these increased. The same trends toward more underreporting than overreporting were observed.

Special Scaling Issues

In the pretest, we included a self-efficacy scale pertaining to efficacy for physical functioning. Thus, for example, items asked how confident the person was that he or she could walk a few blocks or climb a flight of stairs. In the multitrait scaling analyses, items in this efficacy scale correlated equally or more highly with items in the disability scale. Thus, we eliminated the scale from further consideration.

We attempted to develop distinct measures of self-efficacy for managing fatigue and for managing pain and discomfort. However, items correlated highly with one

TABLE 2.9 Correlations Between Self-Efficacy and Corresponding Measures
($N = 140\text{-}478$)

Self-Management Behaviors	
SE exercise regularly:	
with stretching/strengthening exercise	.26
with aerobic exercise	.37
SE get information about disease:	
with use of classes/lectures/support groups	.15
SE obtain help from community, family, and friends:	
with use of tangible resources	.04
with use of classes/lectures/support groups	−.01
with use of organized exercise programs	.09
SE communicate with physician:	
with communicate with physician	.41
Health Status Outcomes	
SE manage shortness of breath:	
with shortness of breath	−.54
SE do social/recreational activities:	
with social/role activities limitations	−.58
with disability	−.36
SE manage symptoms:	
with energy/fatigue	.64
with shortness of breath	−.19
with pain scale	−.41
with pain item	−.42
SE control/manage depression:	
with depressive symptoms (MOS)	−.75
with depression (CES-D)	−.68
with psychological well-being/distress	.72
with health distress	−.49
SE do chores:	
with social/role activities limitations	−.60
with disability	−.51
SE manage disease in general:	
with disability	−.26
with social/role activities limitations	−.42
with depressive symptoms (MOS)	−.55
with depression (CES-D)	−.48
with psychological well-being/distress	.54
with health distress	−.52
with energy/fatigue	.54
with shortness of breath	−.14
with pain scale	−.27
with pain item	−.29

another, thus precluding this possibility. We therefore combined them into an overall measure of self-efficacy for managing symptoms.

In these preliminary studies, we also attempted to develop a measure of limitations in chores and errands as well as a measure of limitations in social and recreational activities. Again, however, the items correlated highly with one another, and the two subscales would not discriminate from each other. Thus, we combined them into an overall social/role activities limitations scale.

With respect to measures of self-efficacy for managing symptoms (fatigue, pain, depression, other symptoms), we initially thought that we could develop distinct constructs pertaining to (a) keeping symptoms from occurring (e.g., keeping from getting tired, depressed) and (b) managing or controlling symptoms once they occurred, as well as keeping symptoms from interfering with the things subjects wanted to do. However, these aspects of self-efficacy for symptom management would not discriminate from one another. Thus, the final scales were a combination of approximately equal questions focusing on both aspects of self-efficacy for managing the symptoms.

Conclusion

We have presented a set of measures that should be useful to investigators attempting to evaluate patient education, health promotion, and other health services interventions. Many of these measures can serve as useful outcomes by which to assess the effectiveness of such interventions. In addition, some of these measures can enable investigators to address the processes by which psychobehavioral interventions are effective in achieving improved outcomes. For example, Lorig and colleagues determined in prior studies of arthritis self-management classes that the improved outcomes were achieved not by changing self-management behaviors but by improving self-efficacy beliefs (Lorig, Seleznick, et al., 1989).

The information in this chapter should be of special interest to those investigating self-efficacy. Subsequent studies that utilize more than one self-efficacy measure should attempt to determine the measures' independence from one another, as well as their independence from the corresponding behavior or outcome.

The measures presented here are intended to be ready to use in their present form. In addition, the methods that we used can serve as a model for developing similar measures for other studies. For example, a nutrition intervention might consider developing self-efficacy measures appropriate to eating habits as well as behavioral measures of actual eating habits.

Some of the measures presented here assess identical constructs (depressive symptoms and CES-D depression). We included these alternative measures to compare their relative usefulness and psychometric characteristics. In selecting a set of outcome measures for a particular study, one would be more likely to select only one measure of each construct. Thus, we would not expect other investigators to include both in a particular study.

The sample on which these measures were developed was substantially more ill on a number of health measures than the MOS sample of patients with one of four chronic conditions (hypertension, diabetes, heart disease, depression) on which many of the health measures were initially developed. This is understandable, given that individuals in this study had enrolled in a chronic disease self-management course and were probably feeling worried about their condition and ill enough to take this course. Thus, it is of particular interest that despite this, the correlations among the measures were quite similar in the two studies. This suggests that samples can vary dramatically in the mean levels of these various constructs but that the measures have an underlying structure (set of relationships among themselves) that is maintained across samples. This is encouraging and supports the application of these measures in diverse populations.

The issue of whether the measures were performing equally well in those with less education or from racial/ethnic minority groups remains to be addressed. Because the sample was highly educated, we could not conduct measurement analyses separately for this group. Such evaluation of the measures is crucial if researchers are to use them in samples with more diversity than is typical.

■ Note

For information on the multitrait scaling program, see Hays and Hayashi (1990) or write to Ron D. Hays, Ph.D., RAND, 1700 Main St., Santa Monica, CA 90407-2138.

■ References

Blalock, S. J., DeVellis, R. F., Brown, G. K., & Wallston, K. A. (1989). Validity of the Center for Epidemiological Studies Depression Scale in arthritis populations. *Arthritis and Rheumatism, 32,* 991-997.

Devins, G. M., & Orme, C. M. (1985). Center for Epidemiologic Studies Depression Scale. In D. J. Keyser & R. C. Sweetland (Eds.), *Test critiques* (Vol. 2, pp. 144-160). Kansas City, MO: Test Corporation of America.

Fries, J. F., Spitz, P., Kraines, R. G., & Holman, H. R. (1980). Measurement of patient outcome in arthritis. *Arthritis and Rheumatism, 23,* 137-145.

Hays, R. D., & Hayashi, T. (1990). Beyond internal consistency reliability: Rationale and user's guide for Multitrait Scaling Analysis Program on the microcomputer. *Behavior Research Methods, Instruments, and Computers, 22,* 167-175.

Likert, R. (1932). A technique for the measurement of attitudes. *Archives in Psychology, 140,* 1-55.

Lorig, K., Chastain, R. L., Ung, E., Shoor, S., & Holman, H. R. (1989). Development and evaluation of a scale to measure perceived self-efficacy in people with arthritis. *Arthritis and Rheumatism, 32,* 37-44.

Lorig, K., Lubeck, D., Kraines, R. G., Seleznick, M., & Holman, H. R. (1985). Outcomes of self-help education for patients with arthritis. *Arthritis and Rheumatism, 28,* 680-685.

Lorig, K., Seleznick, M., Lubeck, D., Ung, E., Chastain, R. L., & Holman, H. R. (1989). The beneficial outcomes of the arthritis self-management course are not adequately explained by behavior change. *Arthritis and Rheumatism, 32,* 91-95.

Mazzuca, S. D. (1982). Does patient education in chronic disease have therapeutic value? *Journal of Chronic Disease, 35,* 521-529.

National Center for Health Statistics. (1991). *The National Health Interview Survey.* Hyattsville, MD: Author.

Nunnally, J. C. (1978). *Psychometric theory* (2nd ed.). New York: McGraw-Hill.

Radloff, L. S. (1977). The CES-D scale: A self-report depression scale for research in the general population. *Applied Psychological Measures, 1,* 385-401.

Ramey, D. R., Raynauld, J. P., & Fries, J. F. (1992). The Health Assessment Questionnaire 1992: Status and review. *Arthritis Care and Research, 5,* 119-129.

Sherbourne, C. D. (1992). Pain measures. In A. L. Stewart & J. E. Ware, Jr. (Eds.), *Measuring functioning and well-being: The Medical Outcomes Study approach* (pp. 220-234). Durham, NC: Duke University Press.

Stewart, A. L., Hays, R. D., & Ware, J. E., Jr. (1988). The Medical Outcomes Study Short-Form General Health Survey: Reliability and validity in a patient population. *Medical Care, 26,* 727-735.

Stewart, A. L., Hays, R. D., & Ware, J. E., Jr. (1992a). Health perceptions, energy/fatigue, and health distress measures. In A. L. Stewart & J. E. Ware, Jr. (Eds.), *Measuring functioning and well-being: The Medical Outcomes Study approach* (pp. 143-172). Durham, NC: Duke University Press.

Stewart, A. L., Hays, R. D., & Ware, J. E., Jr. (1992b). Methods of constructing health measures. In A. L. Stewart & J. E. Ware (Eds.), *Measuring functioning and well-being: The Medical Outcomes Study approach* (pp. 67-85). Durham, NC: Duke University Press.

Stewart, A. L., Hays, R. D., & Ware, J. E., Jr. (1992c). Methods of validating health measures. In A. L. Stewart & J. E. Ware (Eds.), *Measuring functioning and well-being: The Medical Outcomes Study approach* (pp. 309-324). Durham, NC: Duke University Press.

Stewart, A. L., Sherbourne, C. D., Hays, R. D., Wells, K. B., Nelson, E. C., Kamberg, C. J., Rogers, W. H., Berry, S. D., & Ware, J. E., Jr. (1992). Summary and discussion of MOS measures. In A. L. Stewart & J. E. Ware, Jr. (Eds.), *Measuring functioning and well-being: The Medical Outcomes Study approach* (pp. 345-371). Durham, NC: Duke University Press.

Stewart, A. L., Ware, J. E., Jr., Sherbourne, C. D., & Wells, K. (1992). Psychological distress/well-being and cognitive functioning measures. In A. L. Stewart & J. E. Ware, Jr. (Eds.), *Measuring functioning and well-being: The Medical Outcomes Study approach* (pp. 102-142). Durham, NC: Duke University Press.

U.S. Dept. of Health and Human Services. (1995). *Health United States, 1994* (DHHS Pub. No. PHS 95-1232). Hyattsville, MD: National Center for Health Statistics.

Ware, J. E., Nelson, E. C., Sherbourne, C. D., & Stewart, A. L. (1992). Preliminary tests of a 6-item general health survey: A patient application. In A. L. Stewart & J. E. Ware (Eds.), *Measuring functioning and well-being: The Medical Outcomes Study approach* (pp. 291-303). Durham, NC: Duke University Press.

Ware, J. E., Jr., & Sherbourne, C. D. (1992). The MOS 36-Item Short-Form Health Survey (SF-36): I. Conceptual framework and item selection. *Medical Care, 30,* 473-483.

Ware, J. E., Jr., Sherbourne, C. D., & Davies, A. R. (1992). Developing and testing the MOS 20-Item Short-Form Health Survey: A general population application. In A. L. Stewart & J. E. Ware, Jr. (Eds.), *Measuring functioning and well-being: The Medical Outcomes Study approach* (pp. 277-290). Durham, NC: Duke University Press.

Appendixes

Summary and Instructions

These appendixes are organized as follows:

Appendix F: Selected Spanish Language Scales

Appendix G: Sources for More Measures

The instruments presented in these appendixes have been tested. The scales that follow are those that we have found useful, either through our own experience or through the experience of others whose work we admire. Because we cannot present a comprehensive set of instruments here, we have included a list of some other sources that you may find useful in Appendix G.

Each instrument is presented with the scale itself reproduced first. General instructions and the response categories are shown once, rather than with each question as they would be on an actual questionnaire. The individual questions composing the scale are then listed verbatim.

Scoring instructions follow the scales. If the scale's developers have provided instructions on how to handle missing data, we have included them. If not, we generally recommend not scoring the scale if more than 25% of the items are missing. Other authors, however, recommend 50%. Because the missing data cutoff point is arbitrary, you will need to make that decision on the basis of your population and the scale you decide to use.

Following the scoring instructions, we have included a selected bibliography.

Appendix A

Chronic Disease Self-Management Study Measures

LIST OF MEASURES

I. Self-Management Behaviors
Exercise
Cognitive symptom management
Mental stress management/relaxation
Use of community services for tangible help
Use of community services for emotional support
Use of community education and support groups for health problems
Use of organized exercise programs
Communication with physician
Advance directives:
    Has living will/durable power of attorney
    Discussed with doctor
    Discussed with family

II. Self-Efficacy
  1. Self-efficacy to perform self-management behaviors
    SE exercise regularly
    SE get information about disease
    SE obtain help from community, family, friends
    SE communicate with physician
  2. Self-efficacy to manage disease in general
  3. Self-efficacy to achieve outcomes
    SE do chores

SE social/recreational activities
SE manage symptoms
SE shortness of breath
SE control/manage depression

III. Health Outcomes

1. Health status
   Disability
   Social/role activities limitations
   Pain and physical discomfort
   Energy/fatigue
   Shortness of breath
   Psychological well-being/distress
   Depressive symptoms
   Health distress
   Self-rated health
2. Health care utilization
   Visits to physicians
   Visits to mental health providers
   Visits to other providers
   Visits to emergency department
   Hospital stays
   Nights in hospital
   Outpatient surgeries

SELF-MANAGEMENT BEHAVIORS

Exercise

During the past week (even if it was **not** a typical week), how much **total** time (for the **entire week**) did you spend on each of the following? (Please circle **one** number for each question.)

None	Less than 30 minutes/week	30-60 minutes/week	1-3 hours/ week	More than 3 hours/week
0	1	2	3	4

1. Stretching or strengthening exercises (range of motion, using weights, etc.)
2. Walk for exercise
3. Swimming or aquatic exercise
4. Bicycling (including stationary exercise bike)
5. Other aerobic exercise equipment (Stairmaster, rowing or skiing machine)
6. Other aerobic exercise—specify: _____

Note: A validated Spanish translation of this measure can be found in Appendix F.

Scoring. Each category is converted to the following number of minutes spent:

None	Less than 30 minutes/week	30-60 minutes/ week	1-3 hours/ week	More than 3 hours/week
0	15	45	120	180

Time spent in stretching or strengthening exercise is the value for Item 1.
Time spent in aerobic exercise is the sum of the values for Items 2 through 6.

Cognitive Symptom Management

When you are feeling down in the dumps, feeling pain, or having other unpleasant symptoms, how often do you . . . (please circle **one** number for each question)

Never	Almost never	Sometimes	Fairly often	Very often	Always
0	1	2	3	4	5

1. Try to feel distant from the discomfort and pretend that it is not part of your body?
2. Don't think of it as discomfort but as some other sensation, like a warm, numb feeling?
3. Play mental games or sing songs to keep your mind off the discomfort?
4. Practice progressive muscle relaxation?
5. Practice visualization or guided imagery, such as picturing yourself somewhere else?
6. Talk to yourself in positive ways?

Scoring. The score is the mean of the six items. If more than two items are missing answers, set the value of the score for this scale to missing. Scores range from 0 to 5, with a higher score indicating more practice of these techniques.

Mental Stress Management/Relaxation

In the past week (even if it was **not** a typical week), how many **times** did you do mental stress management or relaxation techniques?

[ ] None _____times

Describe what you do to relax: _____

Scoring. Single item only. If technique described is not a cognitive stress management technique, code as "0." Examples of cognitive techniques include progressive muscle relaxation, imagery, prayer, and meditation. Activities such as reading, listening to music, napping, and deep breathing are not considered cognitive strategies and should receive a score of "0." The number of times is then categorized into an ordinal scale with the following categories:

1 = None
2 = 1-7 times/week
3 = 8 or more times/week

This item can also be left as a continuous measure: that is, the actual times per week coded.

Use of Community Services for Tangible Help

In the **past 6 months,** have you gotten help from resources other than friends or family for the following services? (Please circle yes or no for each category.)

	No	*Yes*
Housecleaning	0	1
Yard work	0	1
Home maintenance/repairs	0	1
Meals	0	1
Personal hygiene	0	1
Errands	0	1
Transportation	0	1

Scoring. The score is the count of resources circled "yes," with a possible range of 0 to 7.

Use of Community Services for Emotional Support

In the **past 6 months,** have you gotten help from resources other than friends or family for the following services? (Please circle yes or no for each category.)

	No	*Yes*
Emotional support or counseling	0	1

Scoring. This is a single dichotomous item.

Use of Community Education Services/ Support Groups for Health Problems

Outside of this study, have you attended any classes, lectures, or support groups about your health problem in the **past 6 months?**

[ ] No　　　　[ ] Yes　　　　If yes, how many **total** hours did you attend in the **last 6 months?** _____ hours

Scoring. The score is the hours attended that can then be categorized into an ordinal score with the following categories:

1 = None
2 = 1-5 hours
3 = 6-10 hours
4 = 11 or more hours

This item may also be divided into two separate questions: one asking about attendance at classes or lectures and the other asking about attendance at support groups. The same categorical choices from above can be used.

Use of Organized Exercise Programs

In the **past 6 months,** have you attended any organized exercise programs (such as walking clubs, aerobic classes, or water exercise programs)?

[ ] No   [ ] Yes   If yes, how many **total** hours did you attend
                                 in the **last 6 months?** _____ hours

Scoring. The score is the hours attended that can then be categorized into an ordinal scale with the following categories:

1 = None
2 = 1-18 hours
3 = 19-47 hours
4 = 48 or more hours

Communication With Physician

When you visit your doctor, how often do you do the following? (Please circle **one** number for each question.)

Never	Almost never	Sometimes	Fairly often	Very often	Always
0	1	2	3	4	5

1. Prepare a list of questions for your doctor?
2. Ask questions about the things you want to know and the things you don't understand about your treatment?
3. Discuss any personal problems that may be related to your illness?

Scoring. The score is the mean of the three items. If more than one is missing, set the value of the score for this scale to missing. Scores range from 0 to 5, with a higher score indicating better communication with the physician.

Advance Directives

	(Circle **one**)	
	No	*Yes*
1. Do you have a "living will" or a "durable power of attorney for health matters"?	0	1
2. Have you discussed your wishes in the event of serious illness or impending death with your doctor?	0	1
3. Have you discussed your wishes in the event of serious illness or impending death with your family?	0	1

Scoring. Each question is a single dichotomous item.

SELF-EFFICACY

Self-Efficacy to Perform Self-Management Behaviors

SE Exercise Regularly

We would like to know **how confident** you are in doing certain activities. For each of the following questions, please circle the number that corresponds to your confidence that you can do the tasks regularly at the present time.

How confident are you that you can . . .

Not at all confident	1	2	3	4	5	6	7	8	9	10	Totally confident

1. Do gentle exercises for muscle strength and flexibility three to four times per week (range of motion, using weights, etc.)?
2. Do an aerobic exercise such as walking, swimming, or bicycling three to four times each week?
3. Exercise without making your symptoms worse?

Scoring. Score is the mean of the three items. If more than one item is missing, set the value of the score for this scale to missing. Scores range from 1 to 10, with a higher score indicating greater self-efficacy.

SE Get Information About Disease

We would like to know **how confident** you are in doing certain activities. For each of the following questions, please circle the number that corresponds to your confidence that you can do the tasks regularly at the present time.

How confident are you that you can . . .

Not at all confident	1	2	3	4	5	6	7	8	9	10	Totally confident

1. Get information about your disease from community resources?

Scoring. This is a single-item scale; scores range from 1 to 10, with a higher score indicating greater self-efficacy.

SE Obtain Help From Community, Family, and Friends

We would like to know **how confident** you are in doing certain things. For each of the following questions, please circle the number that corresponds to your confidence that you can do the tasks regularly at the present time.

How confident are you that you can . . .

Not at all											Totally
confident	1	2	3	4	5	6	7	8	9	10	confident

1. Get family and friends to help you with the things you need (such as household chores like shopping, cooking, or transport)?
2. Get emotional support from friends and family (such as listening or talking over your problems)?
3. Get emotional support from resources other than friends or family, if needed?
4. Get help with your daily tasks (such as housecleaning, yard work, meals, or personal hygiene) from resources other than friends or family, if needed?

Scoring. The score is the mean of the four items. If more than one item is missing, set the value of the score for this scale to missing. Scores range from 1 to 10, with a higher score indicating greater self-efficacy.

SE Communicate With Physician

We would like to know **how confident** you are in doing certain activities. For each of the following questions, please circle the number that corresponds to your confidence that you can do the tasks regularly at the present time.

How confident are you that you can . . .

Not at all											Totally
confident	1	2	3	4	5	6	7	8	9	10	confident

1. Ask your doctor things about your illness that concern you?
2. Discuss openly with your doctor any personal problems that may be related to your illness?
3. Work out differences with your doctor when they arise?

Scoring. The score is the mean of the three items. If more than one item is missing, set the value of the score for this scale to missing. Scores range from 1 to 10, with a higher score indicating greater self-efficacy.

Self-Efficacy to Manage Disease in General

SE to Manage Disease in General

We would like to know **how confident** you are in doing certain activities. For each of the following questions, please circle the number that corresponds to your confidence that you can do the tasks regularly at the present time.

How confident are you that you can . . .

Not at all											Totally
confident	1	2	3	4	5	6	7	8	9	10	confident

1. Having an illness often means doing different tasks and activities to manage your condition. How confident are you that you can do all the things necessary to manage your condition on a regular basis?
2. Judge when the changes in your illness mean you should visit a doctor?
3. Do the different tasks and activities needed to manage your health condition so as to reduce your need to see a doctor?
4. Reduce the emotional distress caused by your health condition so that it does not affect your everyday life?
5. Do things other than just taking medication to reduce how much your illness affects your everyday life?

Scoring. The score is the mean of the five items. If more than two items are missing, set the value of the score for this scale to missing. Scores range from 1 to 10, with a higher score indicating greater self-efficacy.

Self-Efficacy to Achieve Outcomes

SE Do Chores

We would like to know **how confident** you are in doing certain activities. For each of the following questions, please circle the number that corresponds to your confidence that you can do the tasks regularly at the present time.

How confident are you that you can . . .

Not at all											Totally
confident	1	2	3	4	5	6	7	8	9	10	confident

1. Complete your household chores, such as vacuuming and yard work, despite your health problems?
2. Get your errands done despite your health problems?
3. Get your shopping done despite your health problems?

Scoring. The score is the mean of the three items. If more than one item is missing, set the value of the score for this scale to missing. Scores range from 1 to 10, with a higher score indicating greater self-efficacy.

SE Social/Recreational Activities

We would like to know **how confident** you are in doing certain activities. For each of the following questions, please circle the number that corresponds to your confidence that you can do the tasks regularly at the present time.

How confident are you that you can . . .

Not at all											Totally
confident	1	2	3	4	5	6	7	8	9	10	confident

1. Continue to do your hobbies and recreation?
2. Continue to do the things you like to do with friends and family (such as social visits and recreation)?

Scoring. The score is the mean of the two items. If either item is missing, set the value of the score for this scale to missing. Scores range from 1 to 10, with a higher score indicating greater self-efficacy.

SE Manage Symptoms

We would like to know **how confident** you are in doing certain activities. For each of the following questions, please circle the number that corresponds to your confidence that you can do the tasks regularly at the present time.

How confident are you that you can . . .

Not at all confident	1	2	3	4	5	6	7	8	9	10	Totally confident

1. Reduce your physical discomfort or pain?
2. Keep the fatigue caused by your disease from interfering with the things you want to do?
3. Keep the physical discomfort or pain of your disease from interfering with the things you want to do?
4. Keep any other symptoms or health problems you have from interfering with the things you want to do?
5. Control any symptoms or health problems you have so that they don't interfere with the things you want to do?

Scoring. The score is the mean of the five items. If more than two items are missing, set the value of the score for this scale to missing. Scores range from 1 to 10, with a higher score indicating greater self-efficacy.

SE Manage Shortness of Breath

We would like to know **how confident** you are in doing certain activities. For each of the following questions, please circle the number that corresponds to your confidence that you can do the tasks regularly at the present time.

How confident are you that you can . . .

Not at all confident	1	2	3	4	5	6	7	8	9	10	Totally confident

1. Keep your shortness of breath from interfering with what you want to do?

Scoring. This is a single-item scale; scores range from 1 to 10, with a higher score indicating greater self-efficacy.

SE Control/Manage Depression

We would like to know **how confident** you are in doing certain activities. For each of the following questions, please circle the number that corresponds to your confidence that you can do the tasks regularly at the present time.

How confident are you that you can . . .

| Not at all confident | 1 | 2 | 3 | 4 | 5 | 6 | 7 | 8 | 9 | 10 | Totally confident |

1. Keep from getting discouraged when nothing you do seems to make any difference?
2. Keep from feeling sad or down in the dumps?
3. Keep yourself from feeling lonely?
4. Do something to make yourself feel better when you are feeling lonely?
5. Do something to make yourself feel better when you are feeling discouraged?
6. Do something to make yourself feel better when you feel sad or down in the dumps?

Scoring. The score is the mean of the six items. If more than two items are missing, set the value of the score for this scale to missing. Scores range from 1 to 10, with a higher score indicating greater self-efficacy.

OUTCOMES

Health Status

Disability

Please circle the one response that best describes your usual abilities over the **past 4 weeks:**

Are you able to . . .

Without any difficulty	*With some difficulty*	*With much difficulty*	*Unable to do*
0	1	2	3

1. Dress yourself, including tying shoelaces and doing buttons?
2. Brush/comb your hair?
3. Stand up from an armless straight chair?
4. Get in and out of bed?
5. Get up from off the floor?
6. Cut your food with a knife or fork?
7. Lift a full cup or glass to your mouth?

AUTHORS' NOTE: The disability section is from "Measurement of Patient Outcomes in Arthritis," by J. F. Fries, P. Spitz, R. G. Kraines, and H. R. Holman, 1980, *Arthritis and Rheumatism, 23,* pp. 137-145. Copyright 1980 by James F. Fries. Adapted with permission.

Without any difficulty	With some difficulty	With much difficulty	Unable to do
0	1	2	3

8. Walk outdoors one block on flat ground?

9. Walk outdoors several blocks on flat ground?

10. Climb up five steps?

11. Climb up one flight of steps?

12. Wash and dry your entire body?

13. Get on and off the toilet?

14. Take a tub bath?

15. Reach and get down a 5-pound object (such as a bag of sugar) from just above your head?

16. Bend down (such as to pick up clothing from the floor)?

17. Open jars which have been previously opened?

18. Turn faucets on and off?

19. Run errands and shop?

20. Do household chores (such as vacuuming, yard work, laundry, and handyman work)?

21. Get to places out of walking distance (by car or public transportation)?

22. Carry a bag of groceries across a room?

Modifications. This is a modified scale based on the Stanford Health Assessment Questionnaire Disability Scale. The following changes have been made:

■ Item 2 replaces "shampoo your hair."

■ Item 5 has been added.

■ In Item 6, "food" replaces "meat."

■ Items 8 and 9 replace one item, "walk outdoors on flat ground."

■ Item 11 has been added.

■ Items 17 and 20 are reworded slightly.

■ Item 21 replaces "run errands and shop."

■ Item 22 has been added.

■ "Open car doors" has been deleted.

■ "Get in and out of a car" has been deleted.

Scoring. There are two ways to score this scale:

1. Score each item independently, such that the score is the mean of the 22 items. If more than 6 questions (or 25%) are missing answers, set the value of the score for this scale to missing. Scores range from 0 to 3, with a higher score indicating more disability.

2. First, score within each category; there are eight categories of items:

   ■ "Dressing and Grooming" includes Items 1 and 2.

   ■ "Arising" includes Items 3, 4, and 5.

- "Eating" includes Items 6 and 7.
- "Walking" includes Items 8, 9, 10, and 11.
- "Hygiene" includes Items 12, 13, and 14.
- "Reach" includes Items 15 and 16.
- "Grip" includes Items 17 and 18.
- "Activities" includes Items 19, 20, 21, and 22.

The score for each category is the response that indicates the greatest degree of difficulty for the items in that category. For example, in the "Dressing and Grooming" category there are responses for two items. If Item 1 ("dress yourself") is marked as "1" and Item 2 ("brush/comb your hair") is marked as "3," then the score for the "Dressing and Grooming" category would be "3," the response indicating the greatest difficulty within that category.

The scale score is the mean of the eight categorical scores. If more than two (or 25%) of the eight categories are missing, set the value of the score for this scale to missing. If fewer than two are missing, then divide the sum of categories by number of existing categories. Scores range from 0 to 3, with a higher score indicating more disability.

Social/Role Activities Limitations

During the **past 4 weeks,** how much . . . (circle one):

Not at all	Slightly	Moderately	Quite a bit	Almost totally
0	1	2	3	4

1. Has your health interfered with your normal social activities with family, friends, neighbors, or groups?
2. Has your health interfered with your hobbies or recreational activities?
3. Has your health interfered with your household chores?
4. Has your health interfered with your errands and shopping?

Scoring. Score is the mean of the four items. If more than one item is missing, set the value of the score for this scale to missing. Scores range from 0 to 4, with a higher score indicating greater limitation in activities.

Pain and Physical Discomfort

1. Please circle the **one** number that best describes your physical discomfort or pain on the **average** over the **past 4 weeks:**

As bad as
None 1 2 3 4 5 6 7 8 9 10 11 12 13 14 15 16 17 18 19 20 **you can imagine**

AUTHORS' NOTE: The pain and physical discomfort section is from *Measuring Functioning and Well-Being: The Medical Outcomes Study Approach,* edited by Anita L. Stewart and John E. Ware, Jr., pp. 373-403. Copyright 1992, RAND Corporation. Reprinted with permission from Duke University Press.

2. Please circle the **one** number that best describes your physical discomfort or pain at its **worst** over the **past 4 weeks:**

                                                               As bad as

None 1 2 3 4 5 6 7 8 9 10 11 12 13 14 15 16 17 18 19 20 **you can imagine**

3. During the **past 4 weeks,** how often have you had physical discomfort or pain? (If you have had more than one discomfort or pain, answer by describing your feelings of discomfort or pain **in general.**) (circle **one**):

> Never 0
> Once or twice 1
> A few times 2
> Fairly often 3
> Very often 4
> Every day or almost every day 5

4. How much bodily discomfort or pain have you generally had during the **past 4 weeks**? (circle **one**):

> None 0
> Very mild 1
> Mild 2
> Moderate 3
> Severe 4
> Very severe 5

5. When you had physical discomfort or pain during the **past 4 weeks,** how long did it usually last? (If you have had more than one discomfort or pain, answer by describing your feelings of discomfort or pain **in general** (circle **one**):

> Didn't have any 0
> A few minutes 1
> Several minutes to an hour 2
> Several hours 3
> A day or two 4
> More than 2 days 5

Modifications. This is a modified version of the MOS pain severity scale, which was changed to omit the skip pattern and add "physical discomfort" to the item stems.

Note: A validated Spanish translation of this measure can be found in Appendix F.

Scoring. To score, first transform each of the five items into a 0 to 100 scale (100 indicating more pain/discomfort), then calculate the mean of the five transformed items. If more than two items are missing, set the value of the score for this scale to missing. Scores range from 0 to 100, with a higher score indicating more pain or physical discomfort.

Energy/Fatigue

These questions are about how you feel and how things have been with you during **the past month.** (For each question, please circle **one** number for **each** question that comes closest to the way you have been feeling.)

How much time during the **past 4 weeks** . . .

None of the time	A little of the time	Some of the time	A good bit of the time	Most of the time	All of the time
0	1	2	3	4	5

1. Did you feel worn out?
2. Did you have a lot of energy?
3. Did you feel tired?
4. Did you have enough energy to do the things you wanted to do?
5. Did you feel full of pep?

Scoring. Items 1 and 3 are reversed as indicated below:

None of the time	A little of the time	Some of the time	A good bit of the time	Most of the time	All of the time
5	4	3	2	1	0

Items 2, 4, and 5 remain unchanged as indicated below:

None of the time	A little of the time	Some of the time	A good bit of the time	Most of the time	All of the time
0	1	2	3	4	5

Reverse Items 1 and 3, then take the mean of the five items. If more than two items are missing, set the value of the score for this scale to missing. Scores range from 0 to 5, with a higher score indicating more energy.

To minimize the number of response sets, items are usually scrambled among other items using the same response categories. This includes items from depression, mental health, and health distress scales.

Bibliography

Stewart, A. L., Hays, R. D., & Ware, J. E., Jr. (1992). Health perceptions, energy/fatigue, and health distress measures. In A. L. Stewart & J. E. Ware, Jr. (Eds.), *Measuring functioning and well-being: The Medical Outcomes Study approach* (pp. 143-172). Durham, NC: Duke University Press.

AUTHORS' NOTE: The energy/fatigue section is from *Measuring Functioning and Well-Being: The Medical Outcomes Study Approach*, edited by Anita L. Stewart & John E. Ware, Jr., pp. 373-403. Copyright 1992, RAND Coporation. Reprinted with permission from Duke University Press.

Shortness of Breath

During the **past 4 weeks,** how much have you been troubled by shortness of breath when doing your normal daily activities? (circle **one**):

Not at all 0
Slightly 1
Moderately 2
Quite a bit 3
Almost totally 4

Scoring. Score is the value of the single item only. Scores range from 0 to 4, with a higher score indicating more shortness of breath.

Psychological Well-Being/Distress
(MOS Mental Health Index III [MHI5])

These questions are about how you feel and how things have been with you during **the past month.** (For each question, please circle **one** number for **each** question that comes closest to the way you have been feeling.)

How much time during the **past 4 weeks** . . .

None of the time	*A little of the time*	*Some of the time*	*A good bit of the time*	*Most of the time*	*All of the time*
0	1	2	3	4	5

1. Have you been a very nervous person?
2. Have you felt downhearted and blue?
3. Have you felt so down in the dumps that nothing could cheer you up?
4. Have you felt calm and peaceful?
5. Have you been a happy person?

Scoring. Items 1, 2, and 3 are reversed as indicated below:

None of the time	*A little of the time*	*Some of the time*	*A good bit of the time*	*Most of the time*	*All of the time*
5	4	3	2	1	0

Items 4 and 5 remain unchanged as indicated below:

None of the time	*A little of the time*	*Some of the time*	*A good bit of the time*	*Most of the time*	*All of the time*
0	1	2	3	4	5

AUTHORS' NOTE: The psychological well-being/distress section is from *Measuring Functioning and Well-Being: The Medical Outcomes Study Approach,* edited by Anita L. Stewart and John E. Ware, Jr., pp. 373-403. Copyright 1992, RAND Coporation. Reprinted with permission from Duke University Press.

First reverse Items 1, 2, and 3, then take the mean of the five items. If more than two items are missing, set the value of the score for this scale to missing. Scores range from 0 to 5, with a higher score indicating better psychological well-being.

To minimize the number of response sets, items are usually scrambled among other items using the same response categories. This includes items from the depression, health distress, and energy/fatigue scales.

Bibliography

Stewart, A. L., Ware, J. E., Jr., Sherbourne, C. D., & Wells, K. B. (1992). Psychological distress/well-being and cognitive functioning measures. In A. L. Stewart & J. E. Ware, Jr., *Measuring functioning and well-being: The Medical Outcomes Study approach* (pp. 102-142). Durham, NC: Duke University Press.

Depressive Symptoms
(MOS Depression/Behavior-Emotional Control)

These questions are about how you feel and how things have been with you during **the past month.** (For each question, please circle **one** number for **each** question that comes closest to the way you have been feeling.)

How much time during the **past 4 weeks** . . .

None of the time	A little of the time	Some of the time	A good bit of the time	Most of the time	All of the time
0	1	2	3	4	5

1. Did you feel depressed?
2. Have you been in firm control of your behavior, thoughts, emotions, and feelings?
3. Did you feel that you had nothing to look forward to?
4. Have you felt emotionally stable?
5. Have you felt downhearted and blue?
6. Have you been moody or brooded about things?
7. Have you been in low or very low spirits?
8. Have you felt so down in the dumps that nothing could cheer you up?

Scoring. Items 2 and 4 are reversed as indicated below:

None of the time	A little of the time	Some of the time	A good bit of the time	Most of the time	All of the time
5	4	3	2	1	0

All other items remain unchanged as indicated below:

None of the time	A little of the time	Some of the time	A good bit of the time	Most of the time	All of the time
0	1	2	3	4	5

First reverse Items 2 and 4, then take the mean of the eight items. If more than two items are missing, set the value of the score for this scale to missing. Scores range from 0 to 5, with a higher score indicating more depression.

To minimize the number of response sets, items are usually scrambled among other items using the same response categories. This includes items from mental health, health distress, and energy/fatigue scales.

Bibliography

Stewart, A. L., Ware, J. E., Jr., Sherbourne, C. D., & Wells, K. B. (1992). Psychological distress/well-being and cognitive functioning measures. In A. L. Stewart & J. E. Ware, Jr. (Eds.), *Measuring functioning and well-being: The Medical Outcomes Study approach* (pp. 102-142). Durham, NC: Duke University Press.

Health Distress

These questions are about how you feel and how things have been with you during **the past month.** (For each question, please circle **one** number for **each** question that comes closest to the way you have been feeling.)

How much time during the **past 4 weeks** . . .

None of the time	A little of the time	Some of the time	A good bit of the time	Most of the time	All of the time
0	1	2	3	4	5

1. Were you discouraged by your health problems?
2. Were you fearful about your future health?
3. Was your health a worry in your life?
4. Were you frustrated by your health problems?

Modifications. This is a modified version of the MOS health distress scale. Only four of six items were used, and the wording of two items was changed. The item "Were you afraid because of your health" was changed to "Were you fearful about your future health," and the item "Were you frustrated about your health" was changed to "Were you frustrated by your health problems."

Scoring. The score is the mean of these four items. If more than one item is missing, set the value of the score for this scale to missing. Scores range from 0 to 5, with a higher score indicating more distress about health.

AUTHORS' NOTE: The health distress section is from *Measuring Functioning and Well-Being: The Medical Outcomes Study Approach*, edited by Anita L. Stewart and John E. Ware, Jr., pp. 373-403. Copyright 1992, RAND Corporation. Reprinted with permission from Duke University Press.

To minimize the number of response sets, items are usually scrambled among other items using the same response categories. This includes items from depression, mental health, and energy/fatigue scales.

Bibliography

Stewart, A. L., Hays, R. D., & Ware, J. E., Jr. (1992). Health perceptions, energy/fatigue, and health distress measures. In A. L. Stewart & J. E. Ware, Jr. (Eds.), *Measuring functioning and well-being: The Medical Outcomes Study approach* (pp. 143-172). Durham, NC: Duke University Press.

Self-Rated Health

In general, would you say your health is . . . (circle **one**):

Excellent	1
Very good	2
Good	3
Fair	4
Poor	5

Note: A validated Spanish translation of this measure can be found in Appendix F.

Scoring. Score is the value of the single item only. Scores range from 0 to 5, with a higher score indicating poorer health.

Bibliography

Idler, E. L., & Angel, R. J. (1990). Self-rated health and mortality in the NHANES-I epidemiologic follow-up study. *American Journal of Public Health, 80,* 446-452.

Schoenfeld, D. E., Malmrose, L. C., Blazer, D. G., Gold, D. T., & Seeman, T. E. (1994). Self-rated health and mortality in the high-functioning elderly: A closer look at healthy individuals. MacArthur Field Study of Successful Aging. *Journal of Gerontology: Medical Sciences, 49,* M109-M115.

U.S. Bureau of the Census. (1985). *National Health Interview Survey.* Washington, DC: U.S. Dept. of Commerce.

Ware, J. E., Jr., Nelson, E. C., Sherbourne, C. D., & Stewart, A. L. (1992). Preliminary tests of a 6-item general health survey: A patient application. In A. L. Stewart & J. E. Ware, Jr. (Eds.), *Measuring functioning and well-being: The Medical Outcomes Study approach* (pp. 291-303). Durham, NC: Duke University Press.

Wolinsky, F. D., & Johnson, R. J. (1992). Perceived health status and mortality among older men and women. *Journal of Gerontology: Social Sciences, 47,* S304-S312.

Health Care Utilization

Visits to Physicians

During the **past 6 months,** did you visit any physician other than a psychiatrist? (Please fill in the blank with a "0" or other number; do **not** include visits while in the hospital.)

How many visits? _____

AUTHORS' NOTE: The self-rated health section is from *Measuring Functioning and Well-Being: The Medical Outcomes Study Approach,* edited by Anita L. Stewart and John E. Ware, Jr., pp. 373-403. Copyright 1992, RAND Corporation. Reprinted with permission from Duke University Press.

Scoring. The score is the count of visits.

Visits to Mental Health Providers

During the **past 6 months,** did you visit any of the following health professionals? (Please fill in the blank with a "0" or other number; do **not** include visits while in the hospital.)

	How many visits?
Psychiatrist	_____
Psychologist or other mental health counselor	_____

Scoring. The score is the sum of the count of these two variables: visits to psychiatrists and psychologists or other mental health counselors.

Visits to Other Providers

During the **past 6 months,** did you visit any of the following health professionals? (Please fill in the blank with a "0" or other number; do **not** include visits while in the hospital.)

	How many visits?
Nurse practitioner or physician's assistant	_____
Home health nurse	_____
Physical, occupational, or respiratory therapist	_____

Scoring. The score is the sum of the count of these three variables: visits to nurse practitioner or physician's assistant, home health nurse and physical, occupational, or respiratory therapists.

Visits to Emergency Room

How many **times** did you visit the **emergency room** in the **past 6 months**?

[ ] None _____ times

Reason for emergency room visit(s): _____

Scoring. The score is the count of times.

Number of Hospital Stays

How many different *times* did you stay in a hospital **overnight or longer** in the **past 6 months?**

[ ] None _____ times

Scoring. The score is the count of times.

Nights in Hospital

How many **total nights** did you stay in a hospital **overnight** in the **past 6 months?**

[ ] None   _____ nights

Reason for hospitalization(s): _____

Scoring. The score is the count of nights.

Outpatient Surgeries

In the **past 6 months,** how many times did you have outpatient surgery (surgery where you did *not* stay overnight in the hospital)?

[ ] None   _____ times

What kind of outpatient surgery did you have?_____

Scoring. The score is the count of times.

Appendix B

Multidimensional Health Profiles

SF-36 HEALTH SURVEY
(MEDICAL OUTCOMES STUDY
36-ITEM SHORT FORM)

INSTRUCTIONS: This survey asks for your views about your health. This information will help keep track of how you feel and how well you are able to do your usual activities.

Answer every question by marking the answer as indicated. If you are unsure about how to answer a question, please give the best answer you can.

1. In general, would you say your health is (circle **one**):

   Excellent 1
   Very good 2
   Good 3
   Fair 4
   Poor 5

2. **Compared to one week ago,** how would you rate your health in general **now**?

[Note to the reader—format the following choices as shown in #1: Much better now than one week ago = 1, Somewhat better now than one week ago = 2, About the same as one week ago = 3, Somewhat worse now than one week ago = 4, Much worse now than one week ago = 5.]

3. The following items are about activities you might do during a typical day. Does **your health now limit you** in these activities? If so, how much? (circle **one** number on each line)

	Yes, limited a lot	*Yes, limited a little*	*No, not limited at all*
a. **Vigorous activities,** such as running, lifting heavy objects, participating in strenuous sports	1	2	3
b. **Moderate activities,** such as moving a table, pushing a vacuum cleaner, bowling, or playing golf	1	2	3
c. Lifting or carrying groceries	1	2	3
d. Climbing **several** flights of stairs	1	2	3
e. Climbing **one** flight of stairs	1	2	3
f. Bending, kneeling, or stooping	1	2	3
g. Walking **more than a mile**	1	2	3
h. Walking **several blocks**	1	2	3
i. Walking **one block**	1	2	3
j. Bathing or dressing yourself	1	2	3

4. During the **past week,** have you had any of the following problems with your work or other regular daily activities **as a result of your physical health**? (circle **one** number on each line)

	Yes	*No*
a. Cut down on the **amount of time** you spent on work or other activities	1	2
b. **Accomplished less** than you would like	1	2
c. Were limited in the **kind** of work or other activities	1	2
d. Had **difficulty** performing the work or other activities (for example, it took extra effort)	1	2

5. During the **past week,** have you had any of the following problems with your work or other regular daily activities **as a result of any emotional problems** (such as feeling depressed or anxious)? (circle **one** number on each line)

	Yes	*No*
a. Cut down the **amount of time** you spent on work or other activities	1	2
b. **Accomplished less** than you would like	1	2
c. Didn't do work or other activities as **carefully** as usual	1	2

6. During the **past week,** to what extent have your physical health or emotional problems interfered with your normal social activities with family, friends, neighbors, or groups?

[Note to the reader—format the following choices as shown in #1: Not at all = 1, Slightly = 2, Moderately = 3, Quite a bit = 4, Extremely = 5]

7. How much **bodily** pain have you had during the **past week**?

   [Note to the reader—format the following choices as shown in #1: None = 1,
   Very mild = 2, Mild = 3, Moderate = 4, Severe = 5, Very severe = 6]

8. During the **past week,** how much did **pain** interfere with your normal work
   (including both work outside the home and housework)?

   [Note to the reader—format the following choices as shown in #1: Not at all = 1,
   A little bit = 2, Moderately = 3, Quite a bit = 4, Extremely = 5]

9. These questions are about how you feel and how things have been with you **during
   the past week.** For each question, please give the one answer that comes closest to
   the way you have been feeling. How much of the time during the **past week** . . .
   (circle **one** number on each line)

	All of the time	Most of the time	A good bit of the time	Some of the time	A little bit of the time	None of the time
a. Did you feel full of pep?	1	2	3	4	5	6
b. Have you been a very nervous person?	1	2	3	4	5	6
c. Have you felt so down in the dumps that nothing could cheer you up?	1	2	3	4	5	6
d. Have you felt calm and peaceful?	1	2	3	4	5	6
e. Did you have a lot of energy?	1	2	3	4	5	6
f. Have you felt downhearted and blue?	1	2	3	4	5	6
g. Did you feel worn out?	1	2	3	4	5	6
h. Have you been a happy person?	1	2	3	4	5	6
i. Did you feel tired?	1	2	3	4	5	6

10. During the **past week,** how much of the time has your **physical health or
    emotional problems** interfered with your social activities (like visiting with
    friends, relatives, etc.)?

    [Note to the reader—format the following choices as shown in #1: All of the time = 1,
    Most of the time = 2, Some of the time = 3, A little of the time = 4, None of the time = 5]

11. How TRUE or FALSE is **each** of the following statements for you? (circle **one**
    number on each line)

	Definitely true	Mostly true	Don't know	Mostly false	Definitely false
a. I seem to get sick a little easier than other people.	1	2	3	4	5
b. I am as healthy as anybody I know.	1	2	3	4	5
c. I expect my health to get worse.	1	2	3	4	5
d. My health is excellent.	1	2	3	4	5

Scoring. The SF-36 has eight subscales: Physical Functioning, Role Limitations Due to Physical Problems, Social Functioning, Bodily Pain, General Mental Health, Role Limitations Due to Emotional Problems, Vitality, and General Health Perceptions. In addition, there is a single-item measure for Reported Health Transition. Scores for each subscale are the sum of the scores for the questions within the subscale. Higher scores mean better health state.

The scores for some questions (1, 6, 7, 8, 9a, 9d, 9e, 9h, 11b, 11d) must be *reversed* before being calculated. (For example, 1 = 6, 6 = 1, 2 = 5, 5 = 2, 3 = 4, 4 = 3)

Subscales are made up of the following items:

Physical Functioning	Items 3a through 3j
Role Limitations—Physical	Items 4a through 4d
Social Functioning	Items 6 and 10 (reverse 6)
Bodily Pain	Items 7 and 8 (reverse both)
General Mental Health	Items 9b through 9d, 9f, 9h (reverse 9d and 9h)
Role Limitations—Emotional	Items 5a through 5c
Vitality	Items 9a, 9e, 9g, 9i (reverse 9a and 9e)
General Health	Items 1, 11a through 11d (reverse 1, 11b and 11d)

The single-item Reported Health Transition is Item 2 (reverse).

If you wish to compare your MOS results with those in other studies using the MOS, you will need to transform the scales. For information on transforming the scales, as well as the handling of missing data, contact the Medical Outcomes Trust, P.O. Box 1917, Boston, MA 02205.

Bibliography

McHorney, C. A., Ware, J. E., Jr., & Raczek, A. E. (1993). The MOS 36-item short-form health survey (SF-36): II. Psychometric and clinical tests of validity in measuring physical and mental health constructs. *Medical Care, 31*(3), 247-263.

McHorney, C. A., Ware, J. E., Jr., Rogers, W., Raczek, A. E., & Rachel Lu, J. F. (1992). The validity and relative precision of MOS short- and long-form health status scales and Dartmouth COOP charts. *Medical Care, 30*(Suppl.), MS253-265.

Stewart, A. L., & Ware, J. E., Jr. (1992). *Measuring functioning and well-being: The Medical Outcomes Study approach.* Durham, NC: Duke University Press.

Ware, J. E., Jr., & Sherbourne, C. D. (1992). The MOS 36-item short-form health survey (SF-36). *Medical Care, 30*(6), 473-483.

ILLNESS INTRUSIVENESS
RATINGS SCALE

The following items ask about how much your illness and/or its treatment interfere with different aspects of your life. PLEASE CIRCLE THE ONE NUMBER THAT BEST DESCRIBES YOUR CURRENT LIFE SITUATION. If an item is not applicable, please circle the number one (1) to indicate that this aspect of your life is not affected very much. Please do not leave any item unanswered. Thank you.

How much does your illness and/or its treatment interfere with your . . .

Not very much   1   2   3   4   5   6   7   Very much

1. Health
2. Diet (i.e., the things you eat and drink)
3. Work
4. Active recreation (e.g., sports)
5. Passive recreation (e.g., reading, listening to music)
6. Financial situation
7. Relationship with your spouse (girlfriend or boyfriend if not married)
8. Sex life
9. Family relations
10. Other social relations
11. Self-expression/self-improvement
12. Religious expression
13. Community and civic involvement

[Use the same response categories for each question.]

Scoring

The Illness Intrusiveness Scale has five subscales:

Physical Well-Being and Diet	Items 1 and 2
Work and Finances	Items 3 and 6
Marital, Sexual, and Family Relations	Items 7, 8, and 9
Recreation and Social Relations	Items 4, 5, and 10
Other Aspects of Life	Items 11, 12, and 13

Average the item scores within each subscale for subscale scores, then average the subscale scores to correct for differences in the numbers of items combined. You may also sum the individual items to generate a total Perceived Intrusiveness score.

AUTHORS' NOTE: *Illness Intrusiveness Ratings Scale,* by Gerald M. Devins, 1981. Copyright 1981 by Gerald M. Devins, Ph.D. Reprinted with permission.

Bibliography

Devins, G. M., Binik, Y. M., Hutchinson, T. A., Hollomby, D. J., Barré, P. E., & Guttmann, R. D. (1983). The emotional impact of end-stage renal disease: Importance of patients' perceptions of intrusiveness and control. *International Journal of Psychiatry in Medicine, 13(4),* 327-343.

Devins, G. M., Mandin, H., Hons, R. B., Burgess, E. D., Klassen, J., Taub, K., Schorr, S., Letourneau, P. K., & Buckle, S. (1990). Illness intrusiveness and quality of life in end-stage renal disease: Comparison and stability across treatment modalities. *Health Psychology, 9(2),* 117-142.

Appendix C

Measures of Individual Health Constructs

MEASURES OF GLOBAL
HEALTH AND QUALITY OF LIFE

General Health Visual Analogue Scale (VAS)

Please mark an "**X**" on the line below to describe your general health in the **recent past.**

Excellent   Poor
    health └——————————————————————————————┘health

Scoring. Measure in centimeters with ruler, "10" being "Poor health" and "0" being "Excellent health." Enter the number where the middle of the "X" is located. Enter whole numbers, not decimals. If the "X" is between centimeters, round down if below 0.5, round up if 0.5 and above, and if exactly at 0.5, round to the nearest even number.

NOTE: The line must be *exactly* 10 cm long. When reproducing, make sure your printer or copy machine reproduces at exactly 100%. You cannot have a reliable measurement if the line is not exactly the same length each time. A small, clear, plastic ruler will make it easier to see the scoring point. Make sure all scoring is done with identical rulers.

Bibliography

Carlsson, A. M. (1983). Assessment of chronic pain. I. Aspects of the reliability and validity of the visual analogue scale. *Pain, 16,* 87-101.

Dixon, J. S., & Bird, H. A. (1981). Reproducibility along a 10 cm vertical visual analogue scale. *Annals of the Rheumatic Diseases, 40,* 87-89.

Downie, W. W., Leatham, P. A., Rhind, V. A., Pickup, M. E., & Wright, V. (1978). The visual analogue scale in the assessment of grip strength. *Annals of the Rheumatic Diseases, 37,* 382-384.

Downie, W. W., Leatham, P. A., Rhind, V. A., Wright, V., Branco, J. A., & Anderson, J. A. (1978). Studies with pain rating scales. *Annals of the Rheumatic Diseases, 37,* 378-381.

Jacobsen, M. (1965). The use of rating scales in clinical research. *British Journal of Psychiatry, 3,* 545-546.

Scott, J., & Huskisson, E. C. (1976). Graphic representation of pain. *Pain, 2,* 175-184.

Scott, P. J., & Huskisson, E. C. (1977). Measurement of functional capacity with visual analogue scales. *Rheumatology and Rehabilitation, 16,* 257-259.

Self-Rated Health

In general, would you say your health is (circle **one**):

```
Excellent  . . . . . . . . . . . . . . . . . .  1
Very good . . . . . . . . . . . . . . . . . .  2
Good . . . . . . . . . . . . . . . . . . . . .  3
Fair  . . . . . . . . . . . . . . . . . . . . .  4
Poor . . . . . . . . . . . . . . . . . . . . .  5
```

For scoring and references, see Appendix A.

Quality of Life Visual Analogue Scale (VAS)

Take a moment and think of the best possible life and the worst possible life. Now, on the line below, place an "**X**" to indicate where your life is now:

Best possible life |———————————————————————| Worst possible life

Scoring. Measure in centimeters with ruler, "10" being "Worst possible life," and "0" being "Best possible life." Enter the number where the middle of the "X" is located. Enter whole numbers, not decimals. If the "X" is between centimeters, round down if below 0.5, round up if 0.5 and above, and if exactly at 0.5, round to the nearest even number.

Note: The line must be *exactly* 10 cm long. When reproducing, make sure your printer or copy machine reproduces at exactly 100%. You cannot have a reliable measurement if the line is not exactly the same length each time. A small, clear, plastic ruler will make it easier to see the scoring point. Make sure all scoring is done with identical rulers.

Bibliography

Carlsson, A. M. (1983). Assessment of chronic pain. I. Aspects of the reliability and validity of the visual analogue scale. *Pain, 16,* 87-101.

Dixon, J. S., & Bird, H. A. (1981). Reproducibility along a 10 cm vertical visual analogue scale. *Annals of the Rheumatic Diseases, 40,* 87-89.

Downie, W. W., Leatham, P. A., Rhind, V. A., Pickup, M. E., & Wright, V. (1978). The visual analogue scale in the assessment of grip strength. *Annals of the Rheumatic Diseases, 37,* 382-384.

Downie, W. W., Leatham, P. A., Rhind, V. A., Wright, V., Branco, J. A., & Anderson, J. A. (1978). Studies with pain rating scales. *Annals of the Rheumatic Diseases, 37,* 378-381.

Jacobsen, M. (1965). The use of rating scales in clinical research. *British Journal of Psychiatry, 3,* 545-546.

Scott, J., & Huskisson, E. C. (1976). Graphic representation of pain. *Pain, 2,* 175-184.

Scott, P. J., & Huskisson, E. C. (1977). Measurement of functional capacity with visual analogue scales. *Rheumatology and Rehabilitation, 16,* 257-259.

MEASURES OF FUNCTION

Health Assessment Questionnaire (HAQ)—Disability Section

Please check (✓) the one response that best describes your usual abilities OVER THE PAST WEEK:

	Without ANY difficulty	With SOME difficulty	With MUCH difficulty	UNABLE to do
Dressing and Grooming				
Are you able to:				
Dress yourself, including tying shoelaces and doing buttons?	☐	☐	☐	☐
Shampoo your hair?	☐	☐	☐	☐
Arising				
Are you able to:				
Stand up from an armless straight chair?	☐	☐	☐	☐
Get in and out of bed?	☐	☐	☐	☐
Eating				
Are you able to:				
Cut your meat?	☐	☐	☐	☐
Lift a full cup or glass to your mouth?	☐	☐	☐	☐
Open a new milk carton?	☐	☐	☐	☐
Walking				
Are you able to:				
Walk outdoors on flat ground?	☐	☐	☐	☐
Climb up five steps?	☐	☐	☐	☐

Please check any **aids or devices** that you usually use for any of these activities:

☐ Cane
☐ Walker
☐ Crutches
☐ Wheelchair
☐ Other (specify:) _____

☐ Devices used for dressing (button hook, zipper pull, long-handled shoe horn, etc.)
☐ Built-up or special utensils
☐ Special or built-up chair

Please check any categories for which you usually need **help from another person:**

☐ Dressing and Grooming
☐ Arising

☐ Eating
☐ Walking

AUTHORS' NOTE: The HAQ disability section is from "Measurement of Patient Outcomes in Arthritis," by J. F. Fries, P. Spitz, R. G. Kraines, and H. R. Holman, 1980, *Arthritis and Rheumatism, 23,* pp. 137-145. Copyright 1980 by James F. Fries. Reprinted with permission.

Please check (✓) the one response that best describes your usual abilities OVER THE PAST
WEEK:

	Without ANY difficulty	*With SOME difficulty*	*With MUCH difficulty*	*UNABLE to do*
Hygiene				
Are you able to:				
Wash and dry your entire body?	☐	☐	☐	☐
Take a tub bath?	☐	☐	☐	☐
Get on and off the toilet?	☐	☐	☐	☐
Reach				
Are you able to:				
Reach and get down a 5-pound object (such as a bag of sugar) from just above your head?	☐	☐	☐	☐
Bend down to pick up clothing from the floor?	☐	☐	☐	☐
Grip				
Are you able to:				
Open car doors?	☐	☐	☐	☐
Open jars that have been previously opened?	☐	☐	☐	☐
Turn faucets on and off?	☐	☐	☐	☐
Activities				
Are you able to:				
Run errands and shop?	☐	☐	☐	☐
Get in and out of a car?	☐	☐	☐	☐
Do chores such as vacuuming and yard work?	☐	☐	☐	☐

Please check any **aids or devices** that you usually use for any of these activities:

☐ Raised toilet seat   ☐ Jar opener (for jars previously opened)
☐ Bathtub seat   ☐ Long-handled appliances for reach
☐ Bathtub bar   ☐ Long-handled appliances in bathroom
☐ Other (specify): _____

Please check any categories for which you usually need **help from another person:**

☐ Hygiene   ☐ Gripping and opening things
☐ Reach   ☐ Errands and chores

Scoring. Each of the eight categories (Dressing and Grooming, Arising, Eating, Walking,
etc.) is coded as a separate unit. The score for each category is determined by the highest
score for **any** of the subquestions in that category.

Without difficulty	*With some difficulty*	*With much difficulty*	*Unable to do*
0	1	2	3

EXAMPLE:

	Without any difficulty	With some difficulty	With much difficulty	Unable to do
	0	1	2	3

Hygiene
Are you able to:

Wash and dry your entire body?	☑	☐	☐	☐
Take a tub bath?	☐	☑	☐	☐
Get on and off the toilet?	☑	☐	☐	☐

This category (Hygiene) would be coded as "1."

Each category is coded according to the basic rules. However, if any "aids or devices" and/or "help from another person" items at the bottom of each page are checked, the score for the category to which they apply is adjusted upward to "2." If the basic score is **already** "2" or "3," the score remains unchanged. "Aids or devices" and "help from another person" can ONLY change a category's score to "2"; they CANNOT change the score to a "1" or a "3."

The categories to which specific devices apply are listed below:

Cane (Walking)
Walker (Walking)
Crutches (Walking)
Wheelchair (Walking)
Bathtub seat (Hygiene)
Bathtub bar (Hygiene)
Long-handled appliance
  for bath (Hygiene)
Other (judge whether it is a
  special device designed for the task,
  not something that is used normally
  by people without disability)

Devices for dressing (Dressing and Grooming)
Built-up or special utensils (Eating)
Special chair (Arising)
Raised toilet (Hygiene)
Jar opener (Grip)
Long-handled appliance for reach (Reach)

Bibliography

Ramey, D. R., Raynauld, J. P., & Fries, J. F. (1992). The Health Assessment Questionnaire 1992: Status and review. *Arthritis Care and Research, 5*(3), 119-129.

MEASURES OF FATIGUE

Multidimensional Assessment of Fatigue (MAF)

These questions are about fatigue and the effect of fatigue on your activities. For each of the following questions, circle the number that most closely indicates how you have been feeling during the past week.

For example, suppose you really liked to sleep late in the mornings. You would probably circle the number closer to the "a great deal" end of the line. This is where I put it:

To what degree do you usually like to sleep late in the mornings?

    1   2   3   4   5   6   7   ⑧   9   10
Not at all   A great deal

Now please complete the following items based on the past week.

1. To what degree have you experienced fatigue? [Format same as #1, with "Not at all" and "A great deal" as anchors.]

   (If no fatigue, please go to Question 17.)

2. How severe is the fatigue which you have been experiencing? [Format same as #1, with "Mild" and "Severe" as anchors.]

3. To what degree has fatigue caused you distress? [Format same as #1, with "No distress" and "A great deal of distress" as anchors.]

Circle the number that most closely indicates to what degree fatigue has interfered with your ability to do the following activities in the **past week.** For activities you don't do, for reasons other than fatigue (e.g., you don't work because you are retired), check the box.

In the past week, to what degree has fatigue interfered with your ability to:

4. Do household chores
Don't do
activity
☐   1   2   3   4   5   6   7   8   9   10
    Not at all   A great deal

   [Items 4-14 are formatted same as #4, with same anchors]

5. Cook

6. Bathe or wash

7. Dress

AUTHORS' NOTE: The MAF is from "Correlates of Fatigue in Older Adults With Rheumatoid Arthritis." Copyright 1993, The American Journal of Nursing Company. Reprinted from *Nursing Research*, March/April, 1993. Used with permission. All rights reserved.

8. Work

9. Visit or socialize with friends or family

10. Engage in sexual activity

11. Engage in leisure and recreational activities

12. Shop and do errands

13. Walk

14. Exercise, other than walking

15. Over the past week, how often have you been fatigued? (circle **one** number)

Every day 4
Most, but not all days 3
Occasionally, but not most days 2
Hardly any days 1
No days 0

16. To what degree has your fatigue changed during the past week?

[Note to the reader—use the same format as #15, with 5 response categories in this order: Increased, Fatigue has gone up and down, Stayed the same, Decreased, I didn't have fatigue this past week]

Scoring. The MAF scale contains 16 items and measures four dimensions of fatigue: severity (Items 1-2), distress (Item 3), degree of interference in activities of daily living (Items 4-15), and timing (Items 15-16).

Do not assign a score to Items 4 through 14 for those respondents who indicated that they "Do not do activity for reasons other than fatigue." If no fatigue on Item 1, assign a zero to Items 2 through 16. Convert Item 15 to 0-to-10 scale by multiplying each score by 2.5. Item 16 is not included in the Global Fatigue Index. To calculate the Global Fatigue Index, sum Items 1, 2, and 3; average of 4 through 14; and newly scored 15.

Bibliography

Belza, B. (1995). Comparison of self-reported fatigue in rheumatoid arthritis and controls. *Journal of Rheumatology, 22,* 639-643.

Note: Users of the MAF are requested to submit the following information for compilation in a database: contact (name, discipline, address, telephone, institution) and research information (study population and projected sample size, research questions driving the measurement of fatigue, and projected time line for data collection and analyses). Mail or fax to Basia Belza, Ph.D., R.N., Department of Physiological Nursing, Box 357266, University of Washington, Seattle, WA 98195-7266; fax 206-543-4711, e-mail basiab@u.washington.edu.

Fatigue Visual Analogue Scale

We are interested in learning whether or not you are affected by fatigue because of your illness. Please mark an "**X**" on the line below to describe your fatigue in the past 2 weeks:

No
fatigue └──┘ fatigue
                                                          Extreme

Scoring. Measure in centimeters with ruler, "10" being "Extreme fatigue" and "0" being "No fatigue." Enter the number where the middle of the "X" is located. Enter whole numbers, not decimals. If the "X" is between centimeters, round down if below 0.5, round up if 0.5 and above, and if exactly at 0.5, round to the nearest even number.

Note: The line must be *exactly* 10 cm long. When reproducing, make sure your printer or copy machine reproduces at exactly 100%. You cannot have a reliable measurement if the line is not exactly the same length each time. A small, clear, plastic ruler will make it easier to see the scoring point. Make sure all scoring is done with identical rulers.

Bibliography

Carlsson, A. M. (1983). Assessment of chronic pain. I. Aspects of the reliability and validity of the visual analogue scale. *Pain, 16,* 87-101.

Dixon, J. S., & Bird, H. A. (1981). Reproducibility along a 10 cm vertical visual analogue scale. *Annals of the Rheumatic Diseases, 40,* 87-89.

Downie, W. W., Leatham, P. A., Rhind, V. A., Pickup, M. E., & Wright, V. (1978). The visual analogue scale in the assessment of grip strength. *Annals of the Rheumatic Diseases, 37,* 382-384.

Downie, W. W., Leatham, P. A., Rhind, V. A., Wright, V., Branco, J. A., & Anderson, J. A. (1978). Studies with pain rating scales. *Annals of the Rheumatic Diseases, 37,* 378-381.

Jacobsen, M. (1965). The use of rating scales in clinical research. *British Journal of Psychiatry, 3,* 545-546.

Scott, J., & Huskisson, E. C. (1976). Graphic representation of pain. *Pain, 2,* 175-184.

Scott, P. J., & Huskisson, E. C. (1977). Measurement of functional capacity with visual analogue scales. *Rheumatology and Rehabilitation, 16,* 257-259.

MEASURES OF PAIN

Gracely Pain

1. Pick the word that best describes the intensity of the strength of your pain in the past 7 days.
   - ☐ Extremely intense
   - ☐ Very intense
   - ☐ Intense
   - ☐ Strong
   - ☐ Slightly intense
   - ☐ Barely strong
   - ☐ Moderate
   - ☐ Mild
   - ☐ Very mild
   - ☐ Weak
   - ☐ Very weak
   - ☐ Faint

2. Pick the word that best describes how bad your pain has been in the past 7 days.
   - ☐ Very intolerable
   - ☐ Intolerable
   - ☐ Very distressing
   - ☐ Slightly intolerable
   - ☐ Very annoying
   - ☐ Distressing
   - ☐ Very unpleasant
   - ☐ Slightly distressing
   - ☐ Annoying
   - ☐ Unpleasant
   - ☐ Slightly annoying
   - ☐ Slightly unpleasant

Scoring. Gracely descriptors are assigned relative magnitude values. Scoring is as follows:

Intensity Scale		Unpleasantness Scale	
Extremely intense	59.5	Very intolerable	44.8
Very intense	43.5	Intolerable	32.3
Intense	34.6	Very distressing	18.3
Strong	22.9	Slightly intolerable	13.6
Slightly intense	21.3	Very annoying	12.1
Barely strong	12.6	Distressing	11.4
Moderate	12.4	Very unpleasant	10.7
Mild	5.5	Slightly distressing	6.2
Very mild	3.9	Annoying	5.7
Weak	2.8	Unpleasant	5.6
Very weak	2.3	Slightly annoying	3.5
Faint	1.1	Slightly unpleasant	2.8

AUTHORS' NOTE: The Gracely pain scales are from "Ratio Scales of Sensory and Affective Verbal Pain Descriptors," by R. H. Gracely, P. McGrath, and R. Dubner, 1978, *Pain, 5,* pp. 5-18. Copyright 1978 by R. H. Gracely. Reprinted with permission.

Bibliography

Gracely, R. H., Dubner, R., & McGrath, P. (1979). Narcotic analgesia: Fentanyl reduces the intensity but not the unpleasantness of painful tooth pulp sensations. *Science, 203,* 1261-1263.

Pain Visual Analogue Scale (VAS)

We are interested in learning whether or not you are affected by pain because of your illness. Please mark an "X" on the line below to describe your pain in the past 2 weeks:

No pain └──┘ Pain as bad as can be

Scoring. Measure in centimeters with ruler, "10" being "Pain as bad as can be" and "0" being "No pain." Enter the number where the middle of the "X" is located. Enter whole numbers, not decimals. If the "X" is between centimeters, round down if below 0.5, round up if 0.5 and above, and if exactly at 0.5, round to the nearest even number.

Note: The line must be *exactly* 10 cm long. When reproducing, make sure your printer or copy machine reproduces at exactly 100%. You cannot have a reliable measurement if the line is not exactly the same length each time. A small, clear, plastic ruler will make it easier to see the scoring point. Make sure all scoring is done with identical rulers.

Bibliography

Carlsson, A. M. (1983). Assessment of chronic pain. I. Aspects of the reliability and validity of the visual analogue scale. *Pain, 16,* 87-101.

Dixon, J. S., & Bird, H. A. (1981). Reproducibility along a 10 cm vertical visual analogue scale. *Annals of the Rheumatic Diseases, 40,* 87-89.

Downie, W. W., Leatham, P. A., Rhind, V. A., Pickup, M. E., & Wright, V. (1978). The visual analogue scale in the assessment of grip strength. *Annals of the Rheumatic Diseases, 37,* 382-384.

Downie, W. W., Leatham, P. A., Rhind, V. A., Wright, V., Branco, J. A., & Anderson, J. A. (1978). Studies with pain rating scales. *Annals of the Rheumatic Diseases, 37,* 378-381.

Jacobsen, M. (1965). The use of rating scales in clinical research. *British Journal of Psychiatry, 3,* 545-546.

Scott, J., & Huskisson, E. C. (1976). Graphic representation of pain. *Pain, 2,* 175-184.

Scott, P. J., & Huskisson, E. C. (1977). Measurement of functional capacity with visual analogue scales. *Rheumatology and Rehabilitation, 16,* 257-259.

MEASURES OF DEPRESSION

Center for Epidemiologic Studies Depression (CES-D)

Below is a list of some of the ways you may have felt or behaved. Please indicate how often you have felt this way during the **past week** by checking (✓) the appropriate space.

Rarely or none of the time (less than 1 day)	Some or a little of the time (1-2 days)	Occasionally or a moderate amount of time (3-4 days)	All of the time (5-7 days)
_____	_____	_____	_____

1. I was bothered by things that usually don't bother me.
2. I did not feel like eating; my appetite was poor.
3. I felt that I could not shake off the blues even with help from my family.
4. I felt that I was just as good as other people.
5. I had trouble keeping my mind on what I was doing.
6. I felt depressed.
7. I felt that everything I did was an effort.
8. I felt hopeful about the future.
9. I thought my life had been a failure.
10. I felt fearful.
11. My sleep was restless.
12. I was happy.
13. I talked less than usual.
14. I felt lonely.
15. People were unfriendly.
16. I enjoyed life.
17. I had crying spells.
18. I felt sad.
19. I felt that people disliked me.
20. I could not get "going."

Scoring

Item Weights	Rarely or none of the time (less than 1 day)	Some or a little of the time (1-2 days)	Occasionally or a moderate amount of time (3-4 days)	All of the time (5-7 days)
Items 4, 8, 12, and 16:	3	2	1	0
All other items:	0	1	2	3

Score is the sum of the 20 item weights. Possible range is 0 to 60. If more than four questions are missing answers, do not score the CES-D. A score of 16 or more is considered depressed.

Bibliography

Radloff, L. S. (1977). The CES-D scale: A self-report depression scale for research in the general population. *Applied Psychological Measurement, 1,* 385-401.

Appendix D

Measures of Health Behaviors

MEDICATION-TAKING MEASURES

Self-Reported Medication-Taking Scale

Please circle "Yes" or "No" for each question:

1. Do you ever forget to take your medicine?	Yes	No
2. Are you careless at times about taking your medicine?	Yes	No
3. When you feel better do you sometimes stop taking your medicine?	Yes	No
4. Sometimes if you feel worse when you take the medicine, do you stop taking it?	Yes	No

Scoring. This scale is designed to test medication compliance. To score, code "Yes" = 0, "No" = 1. The sum of the answers is the score. A score of 4 is considered high compliance, 3 is moderate compliance, and 2 or less is low compliance.

AUTHORS' NOTE: The self-reported medication-taking scale is from "Concurrent and Predictive Validity of a Self-Reported Measure of Medication Adherence," by D. E. Morisky, L. W. Green, & D. M. Levine, 1986, *Medical Care, 24*(1), pp. 67-74. Copyright 1986 by J. B. Lippincott Co. Reprinted with permission.

COPING MEASURES

Coping Strategies Questionnaire

Individuals who experience pain have developed a number of ways to cope, or deal with, their pain. These include saying things to themselves when they experience pain, engaging in different activities. Below are a list of things that patients have reported doing when they feel pain. For each activity, I want you to indicate, using the scale below, how much you engage in the activity when you feel pain, where a "0" indicates you never do that when you are experiencing pain, and a "6" indicates you always do it when you are experiencing pain. Remember, you can use any point along the scale.

Never do			*Sometimes do that*			*Always do that*
0	1	2	3	4	5	6

When I feel pain . . .

_____ 1. I try to feel distant from the pain, almost as if the pain was in somebody else's body.

_____ 2. I leave the house and do something, such as going to the movies or shopping.

_____ 3. I try to think of something pleasant.

_____ 4. I don't think of it as pain but rather as a dull or warm feeling.

_____ 5. It is terrible and I feel it is never going to get any better.

_____ 6. I tell myself to be brave and carry on despite the pain.

_____ 7. I read.

_____ 8. I tell myself that I can overcome the pain.

_____ 9. I count numbers in my head or run a song through my mind.

_____ 10. I just think of it as some other sensation, such as numbness.

_____ 11. It is awful and I feel that it overwhelms me.

_____ 12. I play mental games with myself to keep my mind off the pain.

_____ 13. I feel my life isn't worth living.

_____ 14. I know someday someone will be here to help me and it will go away for awhile.

_____ 15. I pray to God it won't last long.

_____ 16. I try not to think of it as my body, but rather as something separate from me.

_____ 17. I don't think about the pain.

_____ 18. I try to think years ahead, what everything will be like after I've gotten rid of the pain.

_____ 19. I tell myself it doesn't hurt.

_____ 20. I tell myself I can't let the pain stand in the way of what I have to do.

_____ 21. I don't pay any attention to it.

_____ 22. I have faith in doctors that someday there will be a cure for my pain.

_____ 23. No matter how bad it gets, I know I can handle it.

_____ 24. I pretend it is not there.

_____ 25. I worry all the time about whether it will end.

_____ 26. I replay in my mind pleasant experiences in the past.

AUTHORS' NOTE: The coping strategies questionnaire is from "The Use of Coping Strategies in Chronic Low Back Pain Patients: Relationship to Patient Characteristics and Current Adjustment," by A. K. Rosenstiel and F. J. Keefe, 1983, *Pain, 17,* pp. 33-44. Copyright 1983 by Anne Rosenstiel-Gross. Reprinted with permission.

_____ 27. I think of people I enjoy doing things with.

_____ 28. I pray for the pain to stop.

_____ 29. I imagine that the pain is outside of my body.

_____ 30. I just go on as if nothing happened.

_____ 31. I see it as a challenge and don't let it bother me.

_____ 32. Although it hurts, I just keep on going.

_____ 33. I feel I can't stand it any more.

_____ 34. I try to be around other people.

_____ 35. I ignore it.

_____ 36. I rely on my faith in God.

_____ 37. I feel like I can't go on.

_____ 38. I think of things I enjoy doing.

_____ 39. I do anything to get my mind off the pain.

_____ 40. I do something I enjoy, such as watching TV or listening to music.

_____ 41. I pretend it is not a part of me.

_____ 42. I do something active, like household chores or projects.

Based on all the things you do to cope, or deal with, your pain, on an average day, how much control do you feel you have over it? Please circle the appropriate number. Remember, you can circle any number along the scale.

No control			_Some control_			_Complete control_
0	1	2	3	4	5	6

Based on all the things you do to cope, or deal with, your pain, on an average day, how much are you able to decrease it? Please circle the appropriate number. Remember, you can circle any number along the scale.

Can't decrease it at all			_Can decrease it somewhat_			_Can decrease it completely_
0	1	2	3	4	5	6

Scoring. The Coping Strategies Questionnaire has seven subscales, with six items in each subscale, and two single-item effectiveness ratings. To score each subscale, sum the items in each subscale. The higher the score, the more the coping strategy represented by the subscale is used.

The subscales are made up of the following items:

Cognitive coping strategies
    Diverting attention   Items 3, 9, 12, 26, 27, 38
    Reinterpreting the pain sensations   Items 1, 4, 10, 16, 29, 41
    Catastrophizing   Items 5, 11, 13, 25, 33, 37
    Ignoring sensations   Items 17, 19, 21, 24, 30, 35
    Praying or hoping   Items 14, 15, 18, 22, 28, 36
    Coping self-statements   Items 6, 8, 20, 23, 31, 32
Behavioral coping strategy
    Increased behavioral activities   Items 2, 7, 34, 39, 40, 42

Single-item effectiveness ratings are control over pain and ability to decrease pain (last two items).

Appendix E

Patient Satisfaction Measures

PICKER AMBULATORY
CARE PATIENT INTERVIEW

Following are sample questions from the Picker Ambulatory Care Patient Interview. For information about the entire instrument and its scoring, as well as other instruments and workshops developed by the Picker Institute, write to the Picker Institute, 1295 Boylston Street, Suite 100, Boston, MA 02215. This ambulatory care patient interview is from *The Picker Ambulatory Care Patient Interview,* by Margaret Gerteis. Copyright by Margaret Gerteis. Reprinted with permission.

Sample Questions

ACCESS:
    ☐ Were you able to get an appointment as soon as you wanted?
    ☐ If you needed medical advice or help right away, were you able to talk to someone as soon as you needed to?

RESPECT FOR PATIENT PREFERENCES:
    ☐ Did your provider listen to what you had to say?
    ☐ Were you involved in decisions about your care as much as you wanted?

INFORMATION AND EDUCATION:
    ☐ Did you get as much information about your condition and treatment as you wanted from your provider?
    ☐ Did your provider explain why you needed tests in a way you could understand?

☐ When you asked questions, did you get answers you could understand?

EMOTIONAL SUPPORT:
    ☐ Did you have concerns that you wanted to discuss but did not?
    ☐ Did you have confidence and trust in the provider treating you?
    ☐ Did your provider ask you about how your family or living situation might affect your health?

COORDINATION AND CONTINUITY OF CARE:
    ☐ Did your provider explain what to do if problems or symptoms continued, got worse, or came back?
    ☐ Did you have any follow-up visits that you thought could have been avoided by better coordination?
    ☐ Was there ever a time when you thought your doctors did not talk to each other enough about your care?
    ☐ If you were referred to a specialist, did the specialist have the information he/she needed from your medical records?

Scoring. Survey results are reported as problem scores, which are the proportion of patients reporting problems with particular aspects of care. For example, if the patient answers "no" to the question "Did your provider listen to what you had to say?" this is counted as a problem response. The survey includes questions designed to elicit reports about what happened, in addition to questions asking about the patient's satisfaction with care.

GROUP HEALTH ASSOCIATION OF AMERICA (GHAA) CONSUMER SATISFACTION SURVEY

Your Health Care

Thinking about your own health care, how would you rate the following? (circle **one** number on each line)

Poor	Fair	Good	Very good	Excellent
1	2	3	4	5

OVERALL
    1. Overall, how would you evaluate health care at [plan]?

ACCESS: Arranging for and Getting Care
    2. Convenience of location of the doctor's office

AUTHORS' NOTE: The Consumer Satisfaction Survey is from *GHAA's Consumer Satisfaction Survey and User's Manual* (2nd ed.), by A. R. Davies and J. E. Ware, 1991, Washington, DC: Group Health Association of America Inc., Department of Research and Analysis. Copyright 1991 by the Group Health Association of America Inc. Reprinted with permission.

Poor	Fair	Good	Very good	Excellent
1	2	3	4	5

3. Hours when the doctor's office is open
4. Access to specialty care if you need it
5. Access to hospital care if you need it
6. Access to medical care in an emergency
7. Arrangements for making appointments for medical care by phone
8. Length of time spent waiting at the office to see the doctor
9. Length of time you wait between making an appointment for routine care and the day of your visit
10. Availability of medical information or advice by phone
11. Access to medical care whenever you need it
12. Services available for getting prescriptions filled

FINANCES

13. Protection you have against hardship due to medical expenses
14. Arrangements for you to get the medical care you need without financial problems

TECHNICAL QUALITY

15. Thoroughness of examinations and accuracy of diagnosis
16. Skill, experience, and training of doctors
17. Thoroughness of treatment

COMMUNICATION

18. Explanations of medical procedures and tests
19. Attention given to what you have to say
20. Advice you get about ways to avoid illness and stay healthy

CHOICE AND CONTINUITY

21. Number of doctors you have to choose from
22. Arrangements for choosing a personal doctor
23. Ease of seeing the doctor of your choice

INTERPERSONAL CARE

24. Friendliness and courtesy shown to you by your doctors
25. Personal interest in you and your medical problems
26. Respect shown to you, attention to your privacy
27. Reassurance and support offered to you by your doctors and staff
28. Friendliness and courtesy shown to you by staff
29. Amount of time you have with doctors and staff during a visit

OUTCOMES

30. The outcomes of your medical care, how much you are helped
31. Overall quality of care and services

Attitudes Toward Care

Below are some things people say about their medical care. Please read each one carefully, keeping in mind your health care plan. Although the statements may look similar, please answer each one separately. (circle **one** number on each line)

Strongly agree	Agree	Not sure	Disagree	Strongly disagree
1	2	3	4	5

32. I am very satisfied with the medical care I receive
33. There are some things about the medical care I receive that could be better
34. The medical care I have been receiving is just about perfect
35. I am dissatisfied with some things about the medical care I receive

Scoring. For all items except 32 and 34, score as the number circled. Reverse the responses for Items 32 and 34. By using the above scoring, all items and scales are scored with the higher ratings being best.

You have a choice of using the scores for the individual items or to cluster items (as they are in the questionnaire) into a scale (Access, Finances, Technical Quality, Communication, Choice and Continuity, Interpersonal Care, and Attitudes Toward Care). To score a scale add the score of all the items and divide by the number of items in the scale. This will give you the mean or average scale score.

Missing Data: If half or more of the items are missing, consider the whole scale as missing. Do not count missing items when you are figuring a scale score.

Please note: The complete GHAA Consumer Satisfaction Survey contains a number of additional scales for rating one's health insurance plan. The reference for the complete *GHAA's Consumer Satisfaction Survey and User's Manual* (2nd ed.) can be obtained from the Group Health Association of America Inc., Department of Research and Analysis, 1129 Twentieth St. NW, Suite 600, Washington, DC 20036.

Appendix F

Selected Spanish Language Scales

SELF-RATED HEALTH

The following is the Spanish translation of the Self-Rated Health measure found in Appendix A.

    1. Generalmente, Ud. diría que su salud es (Por favor, marque **solamente una** respuesta.)

                  Excelente 1
                  Muy buena 2
                  Buena 3
                  Regular 4
                  Mala 5

For scoring information and selected references, refer to Appendix A.

AUTHORS' NOTE: The following scales were translated and validated by the Stanford Patient Education Research and Arthritis Centers, Palo Alto, CA.

MOS PAIN SEVERITY SCALE

The following is the Spanish translation of the MOS Pain Severity Scale found in Appendix A. This Spanish translation omits the words *physical discomfort* from the item stems and substitutes a 0 to 10 scale of numbered histograms for the original 0 to 20 numeric scale in Items 1 and 2.

1. Por favor marque en la escala el número que mejor describa la intensidad de su dolor en PROMEDIO durante la **última semana:**

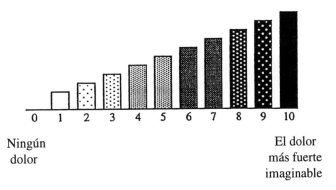

Ningún
dolor

El dolor
más fuerte
imaginable

2. Por favor marque en la escala el número que mejor describa la intensidad de su PEOR dolor durante la **última semana:**

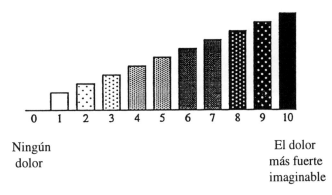

Ningún
dolor

El dolor
más fuerte
imaginable

3. Durante la **última semana,** ¿con qué frecuencia (o qué tan seguido) ha tenido Ud. dolor? (Si ha tenido distintos tipos de dolor, conteste describiendo sus sentimientos de dolor en general.)

Nunca 1
Una o dos veces 2
Pocas veces 3
Seguido (a menudo) 4
Muy seguido (muy a menudo) 5
Todos los días o casi todos los días 6

4. ¿Cómo describiría usted su **dolor del cuerpo** durante la **última semana?**

Ninguno 1
Muy leve (muy suave, muy ligero) 2
Leve (suave, ligero) 3
Moderado 4
Severo (fuerte) 5
Muy severo (muy fuerte) 6

5. Cuando tuvo dolor durante la **última semana,** ¿cuánto tiempo duró normalmente? (Si ha tenido distintos tipos de dolor, conteste describiendo sus sentimientos de dolor en general.)

No tuve ninguno 1
Unos pocos minutos 2
De unos minutos hasta una hora 3
Varias horas 4
Un día o dos 5
Más de dos días 6

For scoring information and selected references, refer to Appendix A.

PAIN VISUAL
ANALOGUE SCALE (VAS)

This is the Spanish translation of the Visual Analogue Pain Scale described in Appendix C. This translation has been slightly modified to read "describe your arthritis pain in the last week," rather then "describe your pain in the past 2 weeks."

1. Estamos interesados en aprender si Ud. está afectado por el dolor a causa de su enfermedad. Por favor marque con una "X" en la línea de abajo para describir su dolor de artritis en la última semana.

Ningún
dolor |_____|

El dolor
más fuerte
imaginable

For scoring information and selected references, refer to Appendix C.

MODIFIED VISUAL
NUMERIC PAIN SCALE

This scale is a modified version of the visual analogue scale for pain developed for the Spanish Arthritis Self-Management Study. The changes include the use of a 0 to 10 numbered scale of histograms instead of the 10-cm line, as well as the additional wording "intensity of your arthritis pain during the last week."

1. Por favor marque en la escala de abajo el número que mejor describa la intensidad de su dolor de artritis durante la **última semana:**

(Please mark on the scale below the one number that best describes the intensity of your arthritis pain during the last week.)

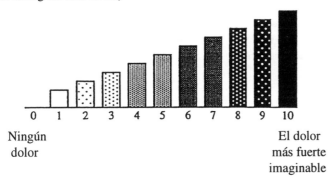

| 0 | 1 | 2 | 3 | 4 | 5 | 6 | 7 | 8 | 9 | 10 |

Ningún
dolor

El dolor
más fuerte
imaginable

Scoring. The score is the number circled or histogram marked. Scores range from 0 to 10, with a higher score indicating more pain.

Bibliography

González, V. M., Stewart, A., Ritter, P., & Lorig, K. (1995). Translation and validation of arthritis outcome measures into Spanish. *Arthritis and Rheumatism, 38,* 1429-1446.

HEALTH ASSESSMENT QUESTIONNAIRE (HAQ)

This is the Spanish translation of the Health Assessment Questionnaire (HAQ) Disability Scale found in Appendix C.

Format of First Page

Por favor marque (✓) la respuesta que mejor describa sus habilidades usuales durante la **semana pasada.**

	Sin ninguna dificultad	*Con alguna dificultad*	*Con mucha dificultad*	*No puedo hacerlo*
¿Actualmente puede Ud:				
Vestirse y arreglarse				
Vestirse, incluyendo amarrarse los zapatos y abrocharse (abotonarse)?	☐	☐	☐	☐
Lavarse la cabeza?	☐	☐	☐	☐
Levantarse				
Levantarse de una silla que no tiene brazos?	☐	☐	☐	☐
Acostarse y levantarse de la cama?	☐	☐	☐	☐

	Sin ninguna dificultad	Con alguna dificultad	Con mucha dificultad	No puedo hacerlo
Comer				
Cortar su comida con cuchillo y tenedor?	☐	☐	☐	☐
Levantar hasta su boca una taza o vaso lleno?	☐	☐	☐	☐
Abrir un cartón nuevo de leche?	☐	☐	☐	☐
Caminar				
Caminar al aire libre en terreno plano?	☐	☐	☐	☐
Subir cinco escalones (gradas)?	☐	☐	☐	☐

Por favor marque cualquier ayuda o aparato que Ud. usa regularmente para estas actividades:

☐ Bastón   ☐ Aparatos o instrumentos para vestirse
☐ Aparato para caminar (andador)   ☐ Utensilios hechos especialmente para Ud.
☐ Muletas   ☐ Silla hecha especialmente para Ud.
☐ Silla de ruedas   ☐ Otro (especifique): _____

Por favor marque las categorías para las cuales necesita regularmente ayuda de otra persona:

☐ Vestirse y arreglarse   ☐ Comer
☐ Levantarse   ☐ Caminar

Format of Second Page

Por favor marque (✓) la respuesta que mejor describa sus habilidades usuales durante la **semana pasada.**

	Sin ninguna dificultad	Con alguna dificultad	Con mucha dificultad	No puedo hacerlo
¿Actualmente puede Ud:				
Higiene				
Bañarse y secarse todo el cuerpo?	☐	☐	☐	☐
Bañarse en la tina del baño (bañadera o bañera)?	☐	☐	☐	☐
Sentarse y levantarse del inodoro (excusado)?	☐	☐	☐	☐
Alcanzar				
Alcanzar y bajar algo que pese 5 libras, de una altura sobre su cabeza?	☐	☐	☐	☐
Agacharse para recoger ropa del piso?	☐	☐	☐	☐
Agarrar				
Abrir la puerta del auto (carro)?	☐	☐	☐	☐
Abrir frascos que ya han sido abiertos?	☐	☐	☐	☐
Abrir y cerrar las llaves del agua (los grifos)?	☐	☐	☐	☐

Actividades
Hacer sus compras? ☐ ☐ ☐ ☐
Subir y bajar del auto (carro)? ☐ ☐ ☐ ☐
Hacer sus tareas domésticas (quehaceres)
o trabajar en jardín? ☐ ☐ ☐ ☐

Por favor marque cualquier **ayuda o aparato** que Ud. usa regularmente para estas actividades:

☐ Asiento elevado para
el inodoro/excusado
☐ Asiento para la tina del baño (bañera)
☐ Agarradera para la tina
del baño (bañera)

☐ Abridor de frascos que han sido
anteriormente abiertos
☐ Aparatos con extensión para alcanzar
☐ Aparatos con extensión para el baño
☐ Otro (especifique): _____

Por favor marque las categorías para las cuales necesita regularmente **ayuda de otra persona:**

☐ Higiene
☐ Alcanzar

☐ Agarrar y abrir cosas
☐ Hacer compras (quehaceres) tareas domésticas

For scoring and selected references, refer to Appendix C.

CENTER FOR EPIDEMIOLOGIC STUDIES DEPRESSION (CES-D)

This is the Spanish translation of the CES-D found in Appendix C.

Lea las frases de abajo que describen cómo se ha sentido o comportado usted **recientemente.**
Por favor marque el número que representa con qué frecuencia se ha sentido de esta manera
durante la última semana.

Raramente o ninguna vez (menos de un día)	*Alguna o pocas veces (1-2 días)*	*Ocasionalmente o una cantidad del tiempo moderado (3-4 días)*	*La mayor parte del tiempo (5-7 días)*
___	___	___	___

1. Me molestaron cosas que normalmente no me molestan.
2. No me sentía con ganas de comer; no tenía apetito.
3. Me sentía que no podía quitarme de encima la tristeza aún con la ayuda de mi familia.
4. Sentía que yo era tan bueno(a) como cualquier otra persona.
5. Tenía dificultad en mantener mi mente en lo que hacía.
6. Me sentía deprimido(a).
7. Sentía que todo lo que hacía era un esfuerzo.
8. Me sentía con esperanza sobre el futuro.
9. Pensé que mi vida había sido un fracaso.
10. Me sentía con miedo.

Raramente o ninguna vez (menos de un día)	*Alguna o pocas veces (1-2 días)*	*Ocasionalmente o una cantidad del tiempo moderado (3-4 días)*	*La mayor parte del tiempo (5-7 días)*
⸺	⸺	⸺	⸺

11. No podía dormir bien.
12. Estaba contento(a).
13. Hablé menos de lo usual.
14. Me sentía solo(a).
15. Pensaba que la gente no era amistosa.
16. Disfruté de la vida.
17. Pasé ratos llorando.
18. Me sentía triste.
19. Sentía que yo no le caía bien (gustaba) a la gente.
20. No tenía ganas de hacer nada.

For scoring information and selected references, refer to Appendix C.

ARTHRITIS SELF-EFFICACY

Below is the Spanish translation of the Arthritis Self-Efficacy (SE) scales, which were modified slightly after psychometric testing to include 6 of the 11 original items for managing pain and other symptoms; this Spanish SE scale also includes 2 new items (Items 3 and 5).

En las siguientes preguntas nos gustaría saber cómo le afecta el dolor de la artritis y qué piensa usted de sus habilidades para controlar su artritis. En cada una de las siguientes preguntas, por favor marque el número que mejor corresponda al nivel de seguridad que siente en este momento de que puede realizar las siguientes actividades.

(In the following questions we would like to know how your arthritis pain affects you and what you think about your abilities to control your arthritis. In each of the following questions, please mark the one number that corresponds best to your level of certainty that you can now perform the following activities.)

1. ¿Qué tan seguro(a) se siente usted de poder reducir bastante su dolor?
   (How certain are you that you can decrease your pain quite a bit?)

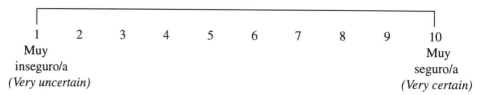

Note to the reader: Insert this scale after each of the following questions.

2. ¿Qué tan seguro(a) se siente usted de poder evitar que el dolor de la artritis no le permita dormir?

   (How certain are you that you can keep arthritis pain from interfering with your sleep?)

3. ¿Qué tan seguro(a) se siente usted de poder evitar que el dolor de la artritis no le deje hacer las cosas que quiere hacer?

   (How confident are you that you can keep the physical discomfort of your arthritis pain from interfering with the things you want to do?)

4. ¿Qué tan seguro(a) se siente usted de poder regular su actividad para mantenerse activo(a) sin empeorar (agravar) su artritis?

   (How certain are you that you can regulate your activity so as to be active without aggravating your arthritis?)

5. ¿Qué tan seguro(a) se siente usted de poder evitar que la fatiga (el cansancio), debido a su artritis, no le permita hacer las cosas que usted quiere hacer?

   (How confident are you that you can keep the fatigue caused by your disease from interfering with the things you want to do?)

6. ¿Qué tan seguro(a) se siente usted de poder ayudarse a si mismo(a) a sentirse mejor si se siente triste?

   (How certain are you that you can do something to help yourself feel better if you are feeling blue?)

7. ¿Comparándose con otras personas con artritis como la suya, ¿qué tan seguro(a) se siente usted de poder sobrellevar el dolor de artritis durante sus actividades diarias?

   (As compared with other people with arthritis like yours, how certain are you that you can manage arthritis pain during your daily activities?)

8. ¿Qué tan seguro(a) se siente usted de poder sobrellevar la frustración debido a su artritis?

   (How certain are you that you can deal with the frustration of arthritis?)

Scoring. The score is the mean of the eight items. If more than two items are missing, set the value of the score for the scale to missing. Scores range from 1 to 10, with a higher score indicating greater self-efficacy.

Bibliography

González, V. M., Stewart, A., Ritter, P., & Lorig, K. (1995). Translation and validation of arthritis outcome measures into Spanish. *Arthritis and Rheumatism, 38,* 1429-1446.

Lorig, K., Shoor, S., & Holman, H. R. (1989). Development and evaluation of a scale to measure perceived self-efficacy in people with arthritis. *Arthritis and Rheumatism, 32,* 37-44.

PHYSICAL ACTIVITIES

This is the Spanish translation of the Chronic Disease Self-Management Study measure for exercise found in Appendix A.

Durante la semana pasada (aún si **no** fue una semana normal) ¿cuánto tiempo en **total** usó (en toda la semana) en cada una de las siguientes actividades?

Ninguno	Menos de 30 minutos por semana	30-60 minutos por semana	1-3 horas por semana	Más de 3 horas por semana
0	1	2	3	4

1. Hacer ejercicio estirar y fortalecer los músculos
2. Caminar como ejercicio
3. Nadar o hacer ejercicios en el agua
4. Andar en bicicleta (incluyendo bicicletas estacionarias)
5. Usar máquinas para ejercicios (como escaleras, remar, etc.)
6. Hacer otro ejercicio aeróbico (especifique): _____

For scoring information, refer to Appendix A.

Appendix G

Sources for More Measures

BOOKS

George, L. K., & Bearon, L. B. (1980). *Quality of life in older persons: Meaning and measurement.* New York: Human Sciences Press.

Kane, R. A., & Kane, R. L. (1981). *Assessing the elderly: A practical guide to measurement.* Lexington, MA: Lexington.

McDowell, I. Y., & Newell, C. (1987). *Measuring health: A guide to rating scales and questionnaires.* New York: Oxford University Press.

Wilkin, D., Hallam, L., & Doggett, M. A. (1992). *Measures of need and outcome for primary health care.* New York: Oxford University Press.

LITERATURE REVIEW ARTICLES

Applegate, W. B., Blass, J. P., & Williams, T. F. (1990). Instruments for the functional assessment of older patients. *New England Journal of Medicine, 322,* 1207-1214.

Wiener, J. M., Hanley, R. J., Clark, R., & VanNostrand, J. F. (1990). Measuring the activities of daily living: Comparisons across national surveys. *Journal of Gerontology, 45,* S229-237.

Index

About the Authors

Virginia González, M.P.H., is Health Educator and Research Assistant at the Stanford Patient Education Research Center in the Stanford University School of Medicine. She received an M.P.H. in health education from the School of Public Health at the University of California, Berkeley, and studied sociology at the University of California, Los Angeles. She has over 9 years' experience collaborating in the development and evaluation of community-based patient educations for people with chronic disease. Currently, she is the coinvestigator on a project to develop and evaluate a culturally relevant Spanish educational program for people with arthritis. She has served as a consultant for community-based organizations, voluntary health agencies, hospitals, and major HMOs in the United States, Canada, and Australia. She also has special interest and skill in working cross-culturally and is the author of a book, articles, and workshops on this topic.

Diana Laurent, M.P.H., is Health Educator and Study Coordinator at the Stanford Patient Education Research Center at the Stanford University School of Medicine. She received her M.P.H. degree at San Jose State University and studied behavioral sciences and communication at the University of California, Davis. She has over 9 years' experience coordinating several research projects at Stanford. She has also served as a consultant for major HMOs, voluntary health agencies, and worksite health promotion organizations in the United States and Canada.

Kate Lorig, R.N., Dr.P.H., is Associate Professor (research) at Stanford University School of Medicine and Director of the Stanford Patient Education Research Center. She has an M.S. in nursing from the University of California, San Francisco, and a Dr.P.H. in health education from the University of California Berkeley School of Public Health. For nearly two decades she has developed and evaluated patient education programs for people with arthritis and other chronic conditions. This work has resulted in more than 40 publications and three books, including *The Arthritis Helpbook, Living a Healthy Life With Chronic Conditions,* and *Commonsense*

Patient Education: A Practical Approach. She has served as a consultant to many groups both in the United States and abroad, including the Veterans Administration Health Education Programs; Kaiser Permanente Health Education Programs; the National Arthritis Foundations of the United States, Australia, and South Africa; and the Arthritis Society of Canada. She has received awards for her work from the National Health Management Foundation, the American Public Health Association, the Society for Public Health Education, and the Arthritis Health Professionals Association.

John Lynch, Ph.D., M.P.H., M.Ed., is Research Epidemiologist at the Human Population Laboratory in Berkeley, California. He earned a Ph.D. in epidemiology and an M.P.H. in health education from the School of Public Health at the University of California, Berkeley. He has been a Wellness Fellow and a National Heart, Lung and Blood Institute Doctoral Fellow, and in 1995 he was the recipient of the Jeremiah Stamler Research Award for New Investigators, which is granted by the Epidemiology and Prevention Council of the American Heart Association. He has more than 10 years' experience in conducting worksite health promotion programs. His major research interests are related to the social patterning of disease. In particular, he has focused on the role of socioeconomic status (SES) as a determinant of health. He has conducted research and written numerous scientific papers on such topics as the role of childhood SES in adult disease; education, income, and occupation as predictors of cardiovascular morbidity and mortality; the relationship of SES over the life course to adult health behaviors; and the impact of job strain on mortality and the progression of atherosclerosis.

Philip Ritter, Ph.D., is Data Analyst for the Chronic Disease Self-Management Study. He was trained in both computer science (B.A., University of California, Berkeley) and anthropology (Ph.D., Stanford University). He conducted anthropological research in Micronesia, where he studied the effects of rapid population growth on family and social organizations. He then became a Research Associate with the Stanford Center for the Study of Families, Children, and Youth, where he remained for over 12 years. His research there included studies of abused and neglected children, families and schooling, and homeless families, and resulted in numerous publications. He has also taught courses in anthropological data analyses and population studies at Stanford. For the past 2 years he has been associated with the Stanford Patient Education Research Center.

Anita Stewart, Ph.D., is Social Psychologist at the Institute for Health and Aging and an Associate Professor in Residence in the Department of Social and Behavioral Sciences, University of California, San Francisco (UCSF). She received her doctorate from the University of California at Los Angeles. She has extensive experience in the conceptualization and measurement of health, health-related quality of life, health behaviors, and other health-related concepts. She was one of the key developers of the Medical Outcomes Study measures of health status while at RAND in Santa Monica prior to joining UCSF. She has published widely on issues in the assessment of health and health-related quality of life in diverse populations. She has served as a consultant to many projects and agencies, including the National Institutes of Health. Her current interests include assessment of health and health-related concepts in a variety of populations and settings, health promotion interventions, aging, and methods for evaluating the effectiveness of health services in minority and disadvantaged populations. She has evaluated the benefits of exercise and physical activity for various populations and recently conducted an intervention to increase the physical activity levels of seniors by encouraging them to participate in physical activity classes and programs offered by the community. She has numerous publications across these diverse areas.